Sure you know the art and science of fitness. But, do you know the business of fitness training? I've seen it a thousand times; Great trainer - Bad business person!

Running a business is not unlike designing a program... You have to understand fundamental business strategies and you have to be able to implement then together into a comprehensive plan for success. Except, your certification curse never taught you that part it!

Put simply, Jon Goodman's book "Ignite the Fire" tells you everything you need to know (and nothing you don't) about how to become successful at the business of Fitness Training. He's provided you with the simple to understand and immediately applicable strategies proven to help you find your niche, how to become the trainer who everyone wants to train with, and how to build a waiting list of clients beating down your door!"

- Nick Tumminello, Owner of Performance University

Jon is passionate about improving the field of personal training. He is visionary in seeing a need for proper high quality personal trainer education. He has applied his knowledge, skills and talent and genuineness and taken a lead in improving his industry.

- Dr. Thomas Ungar, MD, M.Ed, www.mentalhealthminute.com

This is not only some great advices, but rules to live by as a coach/trainer. I have seen myself in what you wrote and how I dealt with it throughout the years and I must say that you did an awesome job. You can be sure that I will refer your work to every trainer, beginner AND advanced, as we tend to forget very simple but so important way of dealing with our clients as we get comfortable in the game. It should be a reference for trainers and coaches to be.

- Eric Falstrault, PICP 5, Owner of BodhiFit

The traditional ways of the personal training industry are gone. Those without business prowess will be swept away or forced to work for someone else. Any personal trainer interested in being their own boss needs to read this, plain and simple. Boom.

- Sam Leahey, Assistant Strength and Conditioning Coach at Springfield College,

Jon's got it nailed. In the complicated world of fitness professional advice, this book is like an arrow on the bullseye. Get it, read it, and start applying. You'll be miles ahead of the competition.

- Paul Valiulis, Precision Nutrition Lean Eating Coach

"This book is exactly what I wish I'd had when I started my career in personal training. This book goes beyond certifications to cover types of employment, client scheduling, marketing, and even business ownership for those who dream of one day running their own facility. Having spent over a decade training people I can say that without a doubt Jon is spot on in his presentation of all elements of this industry. If you aspire to have a successful and exciting personal training career you absolutely must read this book."

- Mark Young, Owner of Mark Young Training Systems

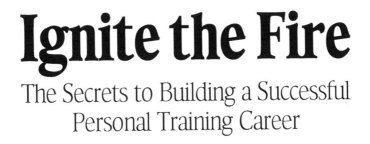

Ignite the Fire

The Secrets to Building a Successful Personal Training Career

by

Jonathan Goodman, CSCS

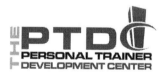

www.theptdc.com

ISBN: 1468168274
ISBN 13: 9781468168273

To my mom and dad

Acknowledgements

Wow! If you'd told me in the winter of 2009 that I would eventually finish this book, I wouldn't have believed you. The day I started, I was up until 4:00 a.m. writing—until I fell asleep in front of my computer (the first of many such occasions!). There were a lot of late nights and long days during the 2 years it took me to complete this book and I have numerous people to thank and acknowledge, not only for helping me with the book, but in my personal and professional journey as well.

The first is my family. My dad has always been my idol and my inspiration. He taught me the value of hard work and always encourages me to critically evaluate any situation. My mom has always been there for me to vent to, and was paramount during the writing process. She was always honest in her critique, which I appreciate—even though I may not have shown it at the time. My sister, Elissa, taught me how to play baseball and instilled in me the love of physical activity. She is now one of my closest friends and is always willing to offer me support. My brother, David, has been my inspiration to be adventurous. He instilled my love of travel when we backpacked through Cuba years ago. My last brother, Daniel, was my closest friend growing up, and I can't thank him enough for always being there for me during all of my impressionable and awkward phases. I love you all.

Second, I want to thank my two best friends, Kyle and Jon. Man, we have been through a lot! I cannot thank both of you enough for your endless support, friendship, guidance, and for lending me your shoulders to lean on when I needed it.

Of course I can't forget my clients, who have taught me more than I could ever hope to teach them. To each of you, thank you. I wouldn't have my career without you.

All of my teachers over the years deserve mention but there is not space here to list all of them. Specifically, however, I am indebted to Dr. Peter Lemon of Western University. Dr. Lemon unknowingly instilled in me a love of physiology and research when he took me into his office for 3 hours to go over the latest creatine and protein studies. Years later, Dr. Lemon took a chance and gave me my first major speaking gig. Teachers like these make a difference, and I am grateful for them.

I've had many mentors, but there are two I'd like to make a special note of. The first is Dr. Adam Martynuik, who took a shy second year kinesiology student and personal trainer and taught him how to lift weights. I credit Adam with showing me the way. Second is Darren Katz, the owner of Body + Soul Fitness in Toronto. Darren developed me as a personal trainer. He pointed me toward good resources, answered my questions, and set me straight when I veered off of my path. I cannot thank him enough and hope to give back even a little bit of what he has given me.

I also owe a big debt of gratitude to my editor, Kelly James-Enger. I still have no idea how she managed to make sense out of 65, 000 words of jumbled nonsense.

My fitness family also deserves a special mention. All of the coaches involved in the Personal Training Development Center (www.theptdc. com) have gone far beyond the call of duty. I owe a massive debt of gratitude to coach Adam Bogar. Without him, the PTDC would not exist. He believed in the vision from the start and helped me make all the initial connections.

Lastly, I want to thank all of my friends and family who I have missed over the last two years. I promise now that this book is out I will return your calls, remember appointments, take a shower, and go out on weekends—at least until I start on the next one…

Table of Contents

Introduction

There's no shortage of books and resources that explain and teach you *how* to become a personal trainer. What's lacking, though, are resources on building a successful, lucrative career in the competitive field of personal training.

In the past, personal trainers have had the reputation of being mindless "muscle monkeys" who lift things up and down for 12 reps and 3 sets. Fortunately that's changing—many personal trainers are as educated as other professionals, and having an exercise science degree is becoming a prerequisite to entering the field.

Successful trainers think critically about everything that they do. They know and understand the reason for different loading regimes and when to use them appropriately. They have enough knowledge of rehabilitation to know when to refer a client to the appropriate professional. And personal trainers know how—and when—to add new equipment to their toolbox.

But that's only the beginning. Personal trainers are now expected to be salespeople, psychologists, nutritionists, post-rehabilitation specialists, and motivational speakers. You can have all of the training expertise in the world, but in order to succeed, you must also be able to inspire passion in your clients, and develop relationships with the people you serve.

That's why I wrote this book. When I became a trainer, I had the exercise and fitness knowledge but I didn't know how to sell myself. I didn't know how to listen to a client. I didn't know how to help a client uncover an emotional reason to exercise. Over time, I learned those essential skills and in just a few years, created a career that exceeded my dreams. Now part of my business is helping personal trainers take their careers to the next level, and this book will help you do that.

My initial drive to write this book, and to create the Personal Trainer Development Center (www.theptdc.com), was to provide resources for personal trainers who may need them. I hope you'll find this book a valuable guide, whether you're new to personal training or want to take a different approach to your work. In the pages that follow you'll find a variety of techniques and strategies to enhance your business. You'll find "Training Tips," which summarize my training philosophies, as well as "Points to Remember" at the end of each chapter. You'll also find "Inside Info," advice from some of the best-known personal trainers in Canada and the U.S. and real-life anecdotes from clients and trainers. (In some cases, names have been changed to protect client privacy.)

I've found personal training to be the most satisfying, exciting, gratifying career in the world. I hope you will find the same to be true, and that this book will help you rise to the challenge of succeeding in this business.

Section 1

Planning for Success

Chapter 1

So, You're a Personal Trainer— What's Next?

"When the student is ready, the teacher will appear."

- BUDDHIST PROVERB

It starts with passion.

Passion is what makes the difference between a successful (and wealthy) personal trainer and one who fails in this business. After seeing countless trainers enter—and leave—this industry, I've analysed what those who make a living, and those who don't, have in common. The biggest factor is a simple one—passion. I mean not only passion for training, but the ability to instil that passion in your clients as well.

Let me explain. Years ago, well-known coach and fitness professional Nick Tumminello classified personal training clients into 3 categories:

1. Performance clients. These clients participate in a sport, whether recreational or professional, and are training to compete at a higher level.
2. Physique clients. These clients want to look great naked. In other words, they're striving to achieve the perfect physical form.
3. Fitness clients. These clients work out for a variety of reasons including stress relief, weight loss, health improvement/maintenance, adding muscle or toning, increased productivity, and enjoyment.

As a personal trainer, the majority of your clients will be fitness clients. These clients don't have the same clearly-defined goals as those in groups 1 and 2. That means they're often teetering on the fence of deciding whether to continue working out with you—or to quit. Advanced loading schemes, periodization, and/or complicated programming will probably not help you keep these clients, irrelevant of how good that programming might be.

Surprised? The fact is that the best and most successful trainers have a good understanding of physiology, anatomy, and biomechanics and they apply their knowledge to workouts. But more importantly, they instil *passion* in their clients every single day. That's what sets them apart.

In the best-selling book, *The Talent Code*, author Daniel Coyle describes what constitutes a great coach for children. The coaches that produce the best athletes from the grass roots level are not the best at teaching skills—they are the best at instilling passion in kids. Walter Gretzky, Wayne Gretzky's father, didn't have the knowledge to address the biomechanics of Wayne's slap shot from a young age. He made Wayne love the game, and that was more important.

Beginning exercisers may not be children, but the same lesson applies. As a trainer, your primary job is not to teach your client to activate their glutes. It's not to have you client perform 3 sets of 12 reps. And it's definitely not to "block-periodize" a training regime. That is the job of physiotherapists, strength and conditioning coaches, and athletic therapists. Your job is to make your client excited to work out and to have him or her love every single workout.

If you're like the vast majority of trainers, more than 90 percent of your clients will be fitness clients. When that's the case, you're not only in the fitness business. You're in the customer service business. The best training regime is the one that will work for each client—and the one that will make clients so happy they keep coming back.

Tuning into your Passion

To help your clients find their own passion, stay tuned into your own. Ask yourself questions like:

- What was your initial motivation for working out?
- How did you start working out? Did you go to a gym? If so, describe the first gym you ever joined in detail.
- What kept you going?
- What obstacles did you face? How did you overcome them?
- At what point did you start to feel successful in the gym? How did that impact your vision of yourself?
- When was the first time somebody noticed the changes in your body? What kinds of comments did you receive? How did that make you feel?
- When was the first time you gave workout advice to somebody else?
- Did your motivation for working out change over time? If so, how?
- What made you decide to make personal training your career?
- What kinds of obstacles did you face to become a personal trainer? How did you overcome them?
- How do you maintain your passion for fitness today?

TRAINING TIP:

Think back to where your passion came from, and work to instil that same feeling in each and every one of your clients. Make them feel what you felt when you made fitness a part of your life and they will stay. When it comes to client retention, passion is more powerful than all of the scientific know-how in the world.

Choosing a Certification

When deciding on which certification is right for you, the first thing to keep in mind is that certifying trainers is a business, and a lucrative one at that. You should decide which certification meshes the most closely with your training philosophy. In addition, different personal training certifications require varying levels of background knowledge and study. Make sure that you're up to the challenge if you decide to apply for a more difficult one but keep in mind that typically the more difficult the certification is to acquire, the more respected it is throughout the industry.

Personal training is unregulated in Canada and the United States. That means that trainers don't have to be certified to work in the industry. However, most gyms' insurance plans won't cover trainers who lack a nationally-recognized certification, and some won't even hire you without one.

The industry has now grown beyond the basic personal trainer. More "side," or additional, certifications are appearing for everything from Kettlebells to older adults specialization to healthy lifestyle coaching. Once again, consider your goals [see chapter 3 for more on developing a training niche] before you sign up for a new certification. Getting certified for the sake of collecting pieces of paper and having letters behind your name may be a waste of money as your clients probably won't know the difference.

What you should keep in mind is that personal training certifications open doors. Can Fit Pro, the Certified Personal Trainers Network (CPTN), and the Canadian Society for Exercise Physiology (CSEP) are all great ways to get started in Canada. In the USA there exists a wider variety of personal training agencies including the American Council on Exercise, the American College of Sports Medicine, and National Academy of Sports Medicine. The benefit of being certified with a large organisation is that they offer workshops, webinars, symposiums, conferences, and other continuing education opportunities to help you further your knowledge.

As a new trainer, I started out with a Can Fit Pro PTS certification, which is a "basic" certification that's relatively easy to obtain. I eventually dropped that certification in favour of the "CSCS" (Certified Strength and Conditioning Specialist) certification offered through the National Strength and Conditioning Association, which is one of the highest-level and most respected certifications available. After doing some research, I found that the CSCS aligned more closely with *my* personal interests than my other certification. The CSCS cert is more oriented toward athletic performance and the monthly research journal I receive is a great resource.

Inside Info – Jonathan Ross

Jonathan Ross is a two-time Personal Trainer of the Year award winner (ACE and IDEA). He's the fitness expert for Discovery Health and the writer of Abs Revealed published by Human Kinetics in 2010.

In 1995 Jonathan's father died from obesity-related blood clots that caused a heart attack. He weighed 424 lbs. His mother was 370lbs. Jonathan knew then that he had found his calling.

He had earned an astronomy degree but had no career aspirations before his father died. He got certified by ACE (in 1997) and started working part time in a health club in the evenings. In January, 2000 he made the jump to a full-time fitness career.

Currently Jonathan trains clients out of a large, multi-purpose health club. He maintains a blog for Discovery Health in addition to providing media expertise for TV, print magazines, and newspapers. He doesn't actively market himself and lets his reputation speak for itself. When clients call they're already sold on his services.

Jonathan's 3 keys to succeeding as a personal trainer are:

1. Take information from others and advance your development by forming your own thoughts, opinions, and training methods – A sure-fire way to spot an intellectually lazy fitness professional is when you hear, "So-and-so says that doing/not doing something is wrong/right." Absolutes are for those lacking the courage to take a balanced perspective.

2. Develop strategies to reach currently under-served markets – The overweight / obese population and the aging population are growing. The obesity numbers are well known and by 2030 it is estimated that 1 in 5 adults in the U.S.A. will be over 65.

3. Be a professional, don't just call yourself one – That means no shirtless photos of yourself on your social media profile or on your website. It's not about you, it's about them. Show your professionalism by your conduct, not your biceps.

Jonathan's words to live by:

"Measure your success by the ability of your clients to follow through on health behaviours when you are not around. Teaching is the process of making yourself unnecessary."

Jonathan Ross is a fitness industry leader and two-time Personal Trainer of the Year award winner (ACE and IDEA). He's also the author of Abs Revealed published by Human Kinetics in 2010. You can find out more at www.absrevealed.com and www. aionfitness.com.

I suggest you take a close look at possible certification organisations before you invest time and money into one. I've compiled a thorough comparison of the different certifications on theptdc.com. Canadians can refer to http://www.theptdc.com/2011/11/top-personal-training-certifications-canada/ and Americans refer to http://www.theptdc.com/2011/11/top-personal-training-certifications-united-states/.

You are your own Advertisement

Walk the walk. If you are a personal trainer, you must be fit and practice what you preach. Think about it. Would you want somebody broke to be investing your money for you? How about getting your hair cut from somebody with a terrible hairdo?

Your physique and your appearance matter. Whether you are in the gym or not, you're a walking advertisement for your product—yourself. I've found most of my clients outside of the gym, either at social events or from conversations with strangers in a coffee shop. Looking fit and appearing professional go a long way in making somebody want to train with you. You never know when you'll meet a potential client—or someone who may pass your name along to a potential client—so you should always be prepared to sell yourself, and hand out business cards.

While working out at the gym, there's a good chance people will notice you. Maybe they'll stare. That's a good thing as your workouts are another form of advertisement. One of the easiest ways to pick up new clients is to work out when your gym is busy. Make yourself visible, leave your headphones off, and put on a show. Performing new or unique-looking variations of exercises may garner questions from interested onlookers which you can use to either build relationships or offer a brief free session or assessment on the spot. Make sure you look approachable and greet people watching you; that may be the opening someone is waiting for to start a conversation with you.

TRAINING TIP:

Always remember you're your own best advertisement, both in and out of the gym. Looking and acting fit is a prerequisite of the job, so behave accordingly.

POINTS TO REMEMBER:

- A successful personal training career starts with passion—the passion you have for your career and your ability to create passion in your clients.

- A fitness certification can help launch your career as a personal trainer, but choose the certification that makes sense for your career.

- As a trainer, you're selling yourself all of the time, sometimes when you least expect it. Make sure you "walk the walk."

Chapter 2

The Right Fit: Finding Work as a Trainer

"Everyone enjoys doing the kind of work for which he is best suited."

- NAPOLEON HILL

Once you've decided on a career as a personal trainer (and likely obtained appropriate certification), you have to decide where you will work. There are lots of opportunities for new trainers starting their careers, and each has advantages and drawbacks. The path you decide to pursue depends on your goals, but this chapter will give you an overview of the variety of places you can work as a trainer. First you'll learn about the most common places for trainers to work, and then about some of the less-popular opportunities.

"Big Box" Gyms

Examples: Bally's, Crunch, Extreme Fitness, Goodlife Fitness, LA Fitness

Working at a "big box" gym is by far the most common path that new trainers choose. These gyms often develop trainers before they move on elsewhere. That being said, many accomplished trainers stay with large organisations for their whole careers. It all depends on your career aspirations.

The push nowadays is for trainers to jump into owning their own facilities, renting space, working as in-home trainers or for smaller clubs, but there are benefits of working at a large gym early on in your career. Yes, sometimes the management of big box gyms mistreat trainers, but there are a number of advantages to starting your career at a large facility. You have access to many clients early on, are able to network, and don't have to worry about the administrative details of running a training business like billing clients and tracking your business expenses. Most large gyms offer trainers access to continuing education through conferences and workshops, and there's definitely a camaraderie that exists in a large gym setting.

Pros
- Marketing ability/power
- Large existing/prospective client base
- Educational opportunities
- Ability to network with other trainers in different areas
- Ability to move up to more senior training positions
- Huge marketing power
- Compensation package can be fair (which may include health insurance)
- Work clothes/uniforms may be provided
- Access to a lot of equipment
- Large offering of services lets you explore different training areas

Cons
- Pay is usually poor
- Management may see trainers as replaceable and mistreat them
- High trainer turnover rates
- Trainers may have unreasonably high sales requirements
- Little care or attention may be given to new trainers
- Driven by profit, not passion

"Boutique" training studios

Example: Body + Soul Fitness (Toronto), Peak Performance (NYC)

The growth of boutique training studios is a relatively new trend but one that is becoming increasingly popular, especially in affluent communities. Boutique studios usually work on an "a la carte" model, allowing clients to choose only the services they want; some do allow clients to purchase "general" memberships. Boutique training studios often focus on higher-end services, attract well-off clients, and tend to be small but quiet and clean.

Pros
- Higher pay than big box gyms
- More personalized management
- Higher end, more dedicated clientele
- Facility tends to be clean and well-appointed
- More access to equipment
- Tends to attract career trainers who are serious about their work

Cons
- Smaller staff means fewer trainers from whom to learn
- Smaller number of current and prospective clients
- Trainers usually must market themselves to attract clients

- May attract clients whose busy schedules interfere with training
- May lack equipment because of smaller size

In-home Training

As people get busier, there's more of a demand for trainers who work at clients' homes. Many new trainers launch their careers as in-home train-ers. As an in-home trainer, you have two options—to work for yourself, as a freelance trainer, or to work for a company (such as Neilson Fitness) as an employee or independent contractor for a company that provides in-home training.

Pros (Freelance)
- No overhead
- Business can be cash-based (but be sure to keep accurate records for taxes)
- Easy to develop a reputation as a neighbourhood trainer
- Can market yourself on a very local basis

Cons (Freelance)
- Must be able to develop your own training systems
- Lack of equipment (unless your client has it)
- Lack of opportunity to learn from other trainers
- Requires constant travel
- Isolation/loneliness
- Solely responsible for marketing yourself and your training business

Pros (Working for a Company)
- Clients are provided for you
- Pay can be competitive
- Training programs are provided
- Company is responsible

Cons (Working for a Company)
- Prohibited from taking on your own clients
- Lack of equipment (unless your client has it)
- Requires constant travel
- Isolation/loneliness

Other Opportunities

Most trainers will work at the four types of training facilities listed above, but there are other training opportunities available too. Those include the following:

"Hardcore" Training Gyms

Example: DeFranco's Training Systems LLC

As the fitness community becomes more segmented, more "hardcore" training facilities are opening up. Generally these are strongman-type operations that use tires, pipes, and sledgehammers in addition to traditional weight-training equipment. These gyms often focus on small group training or boot camp-type sessions as opposed to private, one-on-one training.

Pros
- Strong feeling of loyalty among staff and trainers
- Clientele self-selects this kind of training, so you know what to expect from them
- Group training can be very profitable
- Marketing tends to be handled by the gym

Cons
- Fellow staff members tend to be similar in strengths/ weaknesses
- Focus on specific type of training leaves little room for other styles
- Can be hard to move up

Neighbourhood Community Centers

Many neighbourhood community centers and park districts have fitness centers for residents. In addition to workout equipment, most offer a variety of fitness classes and some now offer personal training. In Canada, some of these positions are salaried government positions; in the U.S., the jobs tend to be hourly ones.

Pros
- May be a salaried position
- Get to be involved with your community
- Opportunity to train those who might not otherwise be able to afford it

Cons
- Pay tends to be low
- Little opportunity to learn from other trainers (you may be the only fitness employee)
- Possible isolation and lack of educational opportunities

Women-only Gyms

Examples: Curves, Women's Workout World

Curves may have been one of the first on the scene, but there are now thousands of women-only gyms throughout Canada and the U.S. (Other gyms offer women-only hours and classes.) Millions of women prefer to work out in a gym that caters to women only, while others have religious beliefs that prevent them from working out in an environment with men.

Pros
- May be a good fit for trainers who want to train women exclusively
- May be the only opportunity for trainers with certain religious beliefs
- Feeling of belonging

Cons

- Gyms may focus on groups exercise (so fewer training opportunities exist)
- Pay rates may be low
- Little variation in training
- Women-only gyms aren't found in some communities

Medical Facilities

Example: MedCan

In the past, medical facilities may have focused on rehabilitative services, but now more medical centers are starting to provide preventive care—and that often means offering fitness centers for patients. Some private medical organisations have full personal training studios (similar to boutique studios) and public hospital fitness programs (particularly pertaining to the bariatric community) are popping up in both Canada and the United States.

Pros

- Opportunity to work with medical professionals in a training facility
- Positions may be contract-based or salaried (so you know what to expect financially)
- Hospitals may offer significant benefits in addition to salary or pay
- Chance to help clients make dramatic and necessary changes
- Opportunity to be part of the growing preventive health care movement

Cons

- Number of facilities is small
- Facilities may be small and not as well-equipped as large gyms
- Facilities may require specific training/background in a medical field

Studio Space

Many privately-owned gyms don't actually hire trainers. Instead, they use a rental model where trainers rent space either by the hour or by the month. Clients may or may not be members of the gym but needn't join the gym to work with a trainer.

Pros
- Can rent space at more than one facility if your clients are spread over a large geographic area
- May have access to a wide selection of equipment
- Small, stable overhead
- Ability to set your own hours and train on your own schedule

Cons
- Responsible for all of your own marketing and promotion
- Responsible for all of your own administrative work
- Quality and type of equipment may vary
- Isolation/lack of other trainers with whom to work and learn

Consider the Inside Track

If you're not sure about a particular position or job opportunity, you may want to consider an internship. Nothing can replace hands-on experience (what may work in a book may not work in real life!), and an internship can give you an opportunity to work with fitness innovators and "big names" in the industry and lead to a paying position at the place you dream of working. Of course, most internships are unpaid, and they require an investment of your time and money that may or may not pay off. Consider how valuable a particular internship would be to you and your career before you pursue one.

If you want to intern somewhere, start with the gym owners or trainers whose work you admire, and ask whether they offer internships. Most of the high-profile gyms have fantastic internship programs but competition to be accepted into one is tough. When you apply for an internship, be sure to mention to the gym owner or trainer *why* you admire him and how his work has influenced you. Go into detail about your future plans within the industry, how you believe he can specifically help you reach your goals, and what you can offer in return.

I suggest you follow up on your application by phone within the first three days. Be persistent. If you are applying for an internship with a well-known trainer (which you should be), I can promise lots of trainers are banging on the same door. You must stand out. Unless the person asks you to stop calling, keep checking in. Your drive may make the difference between being ignored and being offered an internship.

I know some trainers who have gone to outrageous lengths to get internships with top-notch individuals. Take Roger Lawson II, now a highly successful and popular personal trainer. He nabbed a highly coveted internship at Cressey Performance, a Boston training facility famous for producing major league baseball players and numerous books and training materials. Here's his story in his own words:

I knew that I was at a huge disadvantage from the jump because I had a degree in literature and would be going up against people that not only have a degree related to the field, but years of experience on top of that, so I had to stand out.

I found out that Eric [Cressey] was going to be speaking at [Mike] Boyle's annual winter seminar, so I registered, hopped in the car and drove the good ol' twelve hours to Massachusetts to get some knowledge thrown on me as well as to at least make a face-to-face interaction with the CP Staff (this was all before I even graduated, so I still had a few months before applying for the internship). This at least showed them how serious I was and that this wasn't a game to me.

When I applied, I also sent my application next day air, and I made sure to follow up with them every so often about the application progress (not in a pushy way, but often enough so they knew I really wanted it). I did pretty much everything that I could think of to stand out from the applicant pool to compensate for a lack of experience & knowledge.

Roger's approach worked—he got the internship. Since then, "RogLaw," as he is now known, has built a career as a successful personal trainer and a popular Internet fitness personality. (You can find out more about him at www.roglawfitness.com.) Roger didn't just learn how to train during his internship; he also learnt how to build an Internet presence and has used that presence to start a web-based personal training service. Just as important, the internship gave RogLaw the advantage of starting his career as part of the elite's inner circle. As a result, he knows all of the movers and shakers, which has further helped build his career.

If you're serious about an internship, shoot high. You may be surprised that you can launch your career by interning with some of the industry's elite training pros. Well-known trainers and training centers that offer high-quality internships include Michael Boyle (http://www.bodybyboyle.com/); Cressey Performance (http://www.cresseyperformance.com/); and Bill Sonnemaker's Catalyst Fitness (http://www.catalystfitness.com/).

Finding the Right Fit

In today's competitive work environment, your goal is probably simply to find a job. But let me suggest that you choose carefully. Your goal should be to find a position that will provide personal and professional development as well.

To help find the right fit, first decide what type of work appeals to you. You may already have a particular type of position and employer in mind. If not, consider questions like the following:

- Would you rather work for a big or small company?
- What geographic area are you seeking work in? (And are you willing to relocate for a job you really want?)
- What type of clientele do you want to work with?
- What training tools and equipment would you like to have access to?

- What kind of management or supervision would you like?
- What type of space would you like to work in? (Would you rather work in a large facility or a smaller, more intimate setting, for example?)
- How much marketing help do you need? Are you willing and able to market yourself as a trainer?
- Do you need to learn how to close sales with potential clients?
- Are you looking for mentors? What types of mentors would you like to have?
- Do you want to work with other trainers and staff, or would you prefer to work on your own?
- What salary/income are you seeking? What do you need to make to pay your bills?
- What are your long-term goals? For example, what kind of position would you like to have 5 to 10 years from now? Do you want to eventually be a manager, or have your own training business? How will your first job help you reach those goals?

After you've decided what type of work you want to pursue, start your search. You may already have some ideas of where you'd like to apply. *To find other opportunities*:

- Network. Ask friends, colleagues and family members if they know of any great gyms or health clubs that might be hiring. (It's a bonus if they know any employees of these gyms). Tell people you know that you're looking for work and to pass on any ideas to you.
- Start with your certification. Most certification agencies maintain job boards on their websites where you can search for facilities that are hiring.
- Go online. In addition to popular job sites like Monster.com, gyms often use sites like Craigslist, eBay, and Kijiji to post jobs. You can also do a specific Google search for gyms in your area and contact them directly to ask if they're hiring.

You'll need a resume for most training positions, but keep in mind that your resume's job is to get you an interview. It's during the interview that a manager decides to hire you—your skills on paper are nothing compared to how you present them in person.

Use your resume to highlight your relevant qualifications, but streamline your experience. A manager isn't likely to care that you worked at a grocery store during high school or won an achievement award in grade 8. On the other hand, working for the same company for years (which shows loyalty) or winning sports awards in high school or university may be relevant to someone deciding whether to hire you. Make sure you include a section about your personal specialties (for example, low back pain, cardiac rehab), and list the types of clients you are comfortable training, like older adults or pregnant women. And list your certifications and related degrees or other relevant education you've acquired.

Gyms are often in a constant state of hiring, so don't be afraid to contact a gym you want to work for even if they're not actively recruiting. If someone talented applies, they may be hired because managers know that a good trainer will bring in clientele no matter how saturated the market is. In your cover letter, explain why you want to work at that specific gym and what you have to offer.

Inside Info – John Izzo

John Izzo is the owner of Izzo Strength & Performance. He has a packed client list.

In 1998 his job was "supervising the floor" part time at the YMCA while working towards a bachelors degree in public health promotion. Friends, family, and gym members kept asking him questions and he kept researching until he became confident enough to obtain a personal trainer certification.

Since then John has worked for non-profit organisations, commercial facilities, and corporate fitness. He's been a manager at the YMCA, a corporate fitness company, and Gold's Gym.

After 12 years John felt he had enough experience to open his own facility and decided to create an atmosphere that he believed would be conducive to his clients reaching their goals.

John markets mostly through social networks. His blog and facility websites contain resources for exercisers and trainers. Readers spread the word about John's facility through Facebook and Twitter.

John's 3 keys to succeeding as a personal trainer are:

1. Understand where your clients are when they decide to pay for your services – There is an emotional component that brings people to agree to training services and it is up to the personal trainer to harvest a winning attitude from that client.

2. Results are key – Understanding how to apply certain exercise programming specifics for a client is what will bring about adherence and commitment.

3. Create an environment conducive to motivation and support – I can't emphasize enough how important it is to get your clients to start believing that achieving their goals is possible simply by creating a POSITIVE vibe through sessions, consultations, and coaching.

John's words to live by:

"I think it is paramount that trainers step out of this mentality that their job is to "train" or "show exercises". The profession is more about coaching. A trainer has to coach clients to believe and perform better after each session – whether it is attaining new feats of strength, pounds lost, or simply getting them to adjust to newer confidence levels. It is a coaching profession. When you begin to think of yourself as a coach, then you begin to succeed and not accept failure as an option."

John Izzo, NASM-CPT, PES is the owner of Izzo Strength and Performance. He can be found at www.traineradvice.com or www.izzostrengthtraining.com.

The Interview Process

The in-person interview is where you showcase your personality, your knowledge, and your enthusiasm. To prepare for this interview, do as much research on the company as possible and write down possible questions to ask. If you know anyone who works there already, ask him or her about the gym ahead of time.

Dressing appropriately is also important. Even though your work attire will be athletic clothing, you want to look polished. A nice pair of khakis or slacks and collared shirt work well for either gender. Bring copies of your resume and a pad of paper with a pen for taking notes; that shows you're interested and prepared.

From the minute you step foot into the gym, your goal is to make friends. The receptionist may have a lot of power, so don't just flip through a magazine while you wait for your interview. Say hi to the person and get to know him or her a little. (As someone who now hires trainers, I often ask our receptionist her opinion on applicants to see how good they are at "schmoozing.")

Yes, you want a job, but your goal in the interview isn't just to get a job offer. It's to find out whether the gym or facility is a good fit for *you*. Ask questions like:

- What is the main demographic of gym members and/or clients?
- How do sales fit into my role? (Find out whether you're expected to sell a certain number of training hours, for example.)
- Do you have any expectations for billable hours/month? What happens if a trainer doesn't hit them?
- How are you going to market me--and my skills?
- How many trainers do you currently have?
- How many trainers are you currently hiring?
- How long do most trainers stay at your club?
- What programs do you have in place to keep your trainers for the long term?

- How do you monitor your trainers' development?
- How do you monitor training sessions?
- Do you offer support for tasks like greeting clients, following up with clients, and rescheduling appointments?
- Do you have in-house education programs or education funds available for trainers?
- Do you offer mentoring programs for trainers?
- What are the long-term goals of the company?
- What sets your club apart from the competition?

Make sure that the goals and vision of the company align with *your* goals and visions. It's much easier to build a personal training career when you're in the right environment. The most successful trainers are those who take their time, find a great gym that fits their goals, and build their reputation and business from there.

After the interview, make some notes about it while it's still fresh in your mind. If you have multiple interviews or job possibilities, these notes can help you decide which one is the right fit for you. Write down the name of the interviewer (and anyone else you met while there) and consider questions like:

- How well did you connect with the interviewer?
- Can you picture yourself working at the gym?
- Was the overall layout of the gym conducive to your training style?
- Does the organisation's vision and goals align with yours?
- If you met other staff, did you feel that you could work well alongside them?
- What was your overall impression of the staff members you met?
- If you met your potential manager, did you feel you could work well for him or her?
- How did you feel after leaving the interview?
- What did you learn about yourself as a result of the interview?

What to Look For

I had multiple interviews before I accepted the position at the gym where I currently work. After interviewing at different gyms, I realized I wanted a gym that:

- Was small and personal in feel;
- Focused on high-end clientele;
- Employed trainers who used functional training methods;
- Provided me with an opportunity to learn and grow;
- Treated me as an individual and not a number; and
- Would let me play an integral part of a growing organisation.

When I walked through the doors at Body + Soul Fitness, I was immediately greeted by a friendly receptionist. Darren, the owner, walked by and introduced himself, offering me a bottle of water. The club's general manager also introduced herself and chatted with me for a couple of minutes. I immediately felt comfortable, and knew that the environment was right for me.

The sales manager gave me a tour of the facility and answered all of my questions, as well as introducing me to the trainers working on the floor. As the interview went on, I realized that this gym was the perfect fit for me:

- Both employees and clients seemed happy to be there;
- The gym offered an education fund for each trainer in addition to periodic workshops;
- The gym focused on each trainer's unique skills and marketed them accordingly;
- The pay was competitive; and
- The company was planning to expand soon. (In fact, I ended up transferring to the new location when it opened and soon was offered the position of senior trainer there.)

After two more interviews, I was offered the job. I accepted, confident I'd made the right choice. My career has continued to take off since that decision. My point? Know what you're looking for, pay attention during the interview, and make sure that a gym is a good fit for you before you accept a job offer.

Before you say Yes...

So you've been offered a position! Congratulations! Before you say yes, make sure you've taken into consideration the following issues:

- **Hours.** Surprised I didn't list salary or pay first? I cannot stress enough how important it is to know what hours you're expected to work before taking a job. I suggest you decide the amount of hours and days of the week you want to train and don't budge on it. Overworked trainers wind up performing poorly, which is bad for both you and your gym. If the gym has unrealistic expectations for the hours you'll work, it may not be the right place for you. Of course as a new trainer you can expect to work a lot of unpaid hours shadowing other trainers, canvassing the floor, making calls, and marketing yourself in the local community. You'll also spend time waiting for clients; that's part of your job so you want to make the most of those small blocks of time. (I always have a book on me in case a client cancels and I can use a 30-minute break to write up a workout.) At the beginning, remember that spending more hours at the gym early on usually helps you build your clientele more quickly; if you put in fewer hours, you can expect a slower build in clients.
- **Health benefits.** Ask whether a gym offers health benefits; many offer medical and dental coverage and other insurance benefits. This can represent a significant amount of money, especially if you have a family or an existing medical condition.
- **Uniform.** Most gyms require trainers to wear uniforms; they can be as simple as all-black athletic clothing or a shirt with

the gym's logo and khakis. Some gyms have agreements with sports apparel companies that require employees to wear certain brands, so know what you're in for before signing a contract with a gym.

- **Salary.** Salaries for personal trainers range across the board. Certification agencies quote rates from $18-75/hour, with an average hourly rate of about $26/hour. In general, I've found that large gyms tend to offer lower per-hour rates but provide you with clients while smaller gyms offer a higher hourly rate but expect you to do more marketing. Many gyms offer different hourly rates to different levels of trainers. That means that while your initial hourly rate may be relatively low, you can make more by gaining experience. Don't focus only on what you're being offered per-hour but on the overall opportunity. For example, it might be worth it to start at a lower hourly wage in exchange for more support at a gym than take a higher hourly wage at a gym where you wouldn't have as much support and educational opportunities.

Even if you're a new trainer, realize that what is offered salary-wise is probably negotiable. And if you have experience, don't be afraid to ask for a higher hourly rate, or for a commission on sales through the gym, especially if you'll be bringing your current clients with you. Keep in mind that the gym doesn't have to do any marketing to sell to these clients—you've already done that. Second, many clients purchase big packages, which they pay for upfront. That money sits in the gym's bank account accruing interest while you're paid for only one session at a time. I think you're entitled to some of that cash, and many gym managers agree—commissions up to 10 percent of the package price upon initial sale are common.

Before you attempt to negotiate your salary, do some background research and find out what other gyms in the industry are paying trainers with your expertise. Check your certification agency for recent stats or check the website of the International Health, Racquet, and Sportsclub Association (www.ihrsa.org) for salary information. Make sure you understand all of the aspects of your position, and how the gym pays trainers, before you ask for money. Never lie about what you've made in the past, but don't be shy about stating what you want to make—and explaining why you're worth it.

Finally, make sure you're happy with what you'll be making, and excited about working at the gym. Then you've taken the next step to a successful career.

POINTS TO REMEMBER:

- There are many job opportunities for personal trainers, so make sure you understand the pros and cons of each.
- Know what type of job you're looking for before you start your job hunt.
- Focus on finding a position where your personal goals and philosophy align with that of the gym you work at. You'll set the stage for a successful career.

Chapter 3

Set Yourself Apart: Creating your Training Niche

"If you're going to be truly successful, then set yourself apart from everyone else. Go beyond the limits of what classifies the average person and be exceptional."

- DONALD TRUMP

Once you've found work as a trainer, you may think you can simply show up, do your job, and that clients will come to you. And that's true—but to build more than an average career, you have to figure out your training niche. In other words, you don't try to train anyone and everyone. You choose a niche (or more than one) and build your career from there.

After all, the reality is that it is relatively easy to get certified and become a personal trainer. Add to that the fact that anybody in the world can call himself a personal trainer as the industry is unregulated, and you can see that you may have a hard time standing out.

I learned this through practical experience. Early in my career, I was a personal trainer in a boutique gym with a great clientele. I made good money and was helping my clients obtain results, but I still felt unfulfilled. Fortunately a mentor gave me what I thought was the ultra-secret two-step method to success:

1. Do a great job.

2. Make sure everybody knows about it.

Once I put this "secret" into action, I began building a reputation as an expert—first locally, nationally, and eventually internationally. The easiest way to do so is to choose a training niche and become an expert about it. I knew that I loved the "softer" side of personal training—motivating, teaching, and inspiring clients. While I knew a lot about exercise prescription, I wasn't as interested in that aspect of training. I decided to diligently research the often-ignored "softer" aspects of personal training and created my niche.

There's nothing wrong with being an average trainer or for settling for an average career. If you want to stand out, though, you must become an expert in one particular type of training. Pick something you're passionate about and run with it.

What makes you different?

Once you've decided what your niche will be, you have to market your specific skills to your clients and the public. Eventually when people think of that niche, they should think of you, and vice-versa.

Take the well-known coaches, Eric Cressey and Bret Contreras. Each built his name and reputation by focusing on one specific type of training. Eric Cressey is best known for shoulder performance (and as a result, training baseball players) and Bret Contreras is known to all in the fitness arena as the "glute guy."

Do Cressey and Contreras train solely within their specialty? Absolutely not! But they both recognized that in order to build up a reputation, they had to pick one aspect of training and become the go-to guy on that subject. Once each had established his reputation, he was free to explore other specialities.

I encourage you to take the same approach with the people you train, and with the people you encounter. The path you take depends on your long-term goals within the industry. If you want to eventually stand out on the international or national scale, follow Cressey's or Contreras' path, choose a type of training that few people are focusing on, and do your research. It takes time and dedication to build up a strong knowledge base.

Even if your goal isn't as lofty as becoming internationally recognized, I still encourage you to create a training niche. Think about your clients' needs and look at areas in which you can specialize. For example, chronic low back pain is a major source of discomfort and even debilitating pain for many people. However, most trainers can help clients address low back pain relatively quickly once they learn how to perform muscle imbalance testing and become familiar with the work of professionals like exercise kinesiology expert Paul Chek and lower back pain expert Dr. Stu McGill.

Look at your clients and potential clients with an inquisitive eye. Are they professionals who all suffer from low back pain and bad posture? Do you train a lot of older adults who require balance and functional training? Maybe there are a lot of young mothers at the gym who would be interested in prenatal and postnatal training.

I suggest you consider two primary needs in your target clientele (for example, low back pain, weight loss, preventing or managing diabetes, or gaining muscle). Once you've identified those needs, determine whether anyone else is currently serving people with them. If other trainers or professionals are specializing in these clients, can you team up with those providers—or provide better service to their target clients?

Consider too whether there are clients who have needs that aren't being served. Let's say you live in a community that has a large number of people with diabetes, yet no trainers specialize in training people with the disease. Are there other types of clients with specific challenges you could work with? List those potential clients and their needs, and then determine how you can serve them if you're not already in a position to do so.

That might include:

- Attaining more education about those specific needs;
- Attaining additional certifications;
- Connecting with charities that serve these people;
- Connecting with professionals in different fields that serve the same population (for example, registered dieticians or athletic trainers);
- Marketing specifically to the target clients; and
- Asking your current clients if they know people with these needs. (Have a handout ready to give to your client so they can pass it on to their friend.)

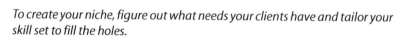

TRAINING TIP:

To create your niche, figure out what needs your clients have and tailor your skill set to fill the holes.

Inside Info – Bret Contreras

Bret Contreras is known as the Glute Guy in internet circles and has built up a reputation through studying and designing programs for peoples' backsides.

Bret received his first personal training certification at 21, but had been training friends and family members long before then. Bret opened *Lifts Studio* in Scottsdale Arizona. Being an obsessive researcher, he conducted hundreds of Electromyography (EMG) experiments. He invented the *Scorcher* (a glutes strengthening machine) and wrote *Advanced Techniques in Glutei Maximi Strengthening.*

Bret has trained clients in large commercial gyms, personal training studios, garage gyms, parks, and in-home. His business has always been based on referrals and his blog.

At the time of publication Bret has only two personal and six online training clients. He is pursuing his PhD in New Zealand and writing two books.

Bret's 3 keys to succeeding as a personal trainer are:

1. Work out and achieve satisfactory results – You must practice what you preach.

2. Read and continue to learn – Blogs, websites, magazines, journals, textbooks, courses, and seminars all work. There is a ton of information out there; it's up to you to make use of it.

3. Be dependable, motivating, and sincere – If you don't care about your clients results you've chosen the wrong career.

Bret's words to live by:

"One of the most critical components to achieving success is learning proper movement patterns. Become a master of exercise form. If your clients can squat, lunge, hip hinge, push up, chin, row, bridge, and plank properly, then they're already leaps and bounds above the majority of individuals."

Bret Contreras MA, CSCS is currently completing his PhD in New Zealand and is writing two books for publication. You can read his blog at www.bretcontreras.com

Spread the Word

Once you've chosen your niche, it is time to let the world (or at least your neighbourhood) know. Here are several effective ways to get the word out about your new speciality:

- **Master your two-sentence pitch.** In other words, you must be able to explain to potential clients what makes you different in two sentences. If you can't talk about it succinctly, no one else can either.
- **Write.** Most well-known trainers have blogs they maintain, and I do recommend a blog if you can afford the time to post at least once or twice a week. Even if you don't blog, you still should create a short handout about your speciality. Brand it with your (or your company's) logo and provide some valuable information about the subject of your niche. For example, if you want to specialize in lower back training, your handout might explain why lower back pain is so common, citing recent research. Give copies to your clients to distribute.
- **Speak.** Offer a free workshop to your clients and potential clients on one aspect of your niche. Advertise it in local coffee shops, at the gym, and with flyers in local stores, and ask your clients to help spread the word. These workshops are not only a way to meet potential new clients but also give existing clients a chance to know each other, strengthening your professional community.
- **Do a great job.** The most effective marketing technique is producing results for your clients. Build a strong, positive relationship with each client you work with, and help them achieve their goals. If you can't help them with a particular issue, refer them to someone who can. And always remember to ask for referrals. When you do a great job for people, your current clients are always your biggest source of new clients.

TRAINING TIP:

Once you've created your niche, make sure that everyone knows about it.

Setting yourself Apart: A Case Study

Remember that any potential client has dozens, if not hundreds of trainers, from whom to choose. You can't try to be everything to everybody—that is a recipe for an average career. To stand out, figure out what your niche is, and stick to it.

For example, when Body + Soul Fitness decided to open a second location in midtown Toronto in 2007, the studio was less than a 10-minute walk from 3 big box gyms. Body + Soul's stated purpose was to provide a more personal feel and high quality personal training environment than the big gyms did, but it failed initially.

The first 2 years, Body + Soul tried to be everything to everyone. (And you know now that's impossible!) While its initial mission may have been to provide a more personal approach, the focus soon became gaining members. The club offered discounts, sent a mass mailing to 30,000 local homes, and altered its group exercise schedule monthly to try to attract members.

But Body + Soul Fitness is not a big gym, and its marketing budget was small. The mass mailing was expensive, yet failed to pull in new clients. And offering group exercise classes was expensive, yet drew few participants who were interested in personal training. It wasn't until Body + Soul's management decided to focus on what it could do better than its big box competitors that it started to thrive. Its competitive advantage was personal training.

The neighbourhood leaders had their primary strength in numbers. They were all large gyms that offered cheap memberships and had full group exercise programs and lots of equipment. However, the big gyms' weakness was the lack of personal attention paid to members. Body + Soul focused on hiring and retaining highly qualified trainers who specialized in different niches and who gave one-on-one attention to their clients. To help spread the word, the gym also identified the "mavens" in the area, and offered them free memberships. (Author Malcolm Gladwell describes "mavens" in his bestseller, *The Tipping Point*, as those who have the power to influence large groups of people. His book is a worthwhile read if you want to know more about how to connect with people who can help you build and promote your personal training business.)

In this case the mavens were the people in the neighbourhood who had the power to influence many others. They were intelligent, well respected, and had jobs where they interacted with lots of people (think real estate agents, doctors, and local shop and business owners). These mavens comprised more marketing power than any mailing campaign could dream of, and in less than a year Body + Soul was thriving and profitable. The key was proper positioning.

My point? In today's market, you must position yourself to stand out and be successful. Creating a niche and spreading the word about it will help you do that.

POINTS TO REMEMBER:

- To stand out, you must create a niche for yourself.
- To determine your niche, determine what need your clients and potential clients have that are not being met, and focus on them.
- Once you have your niche, continually communicate it to the people around you.

Section 2

Working as a Personal Trainer

Chapter 4

You're in Sales Now:
The Art of Selling

"I find it useful to remember everyone lives by selling something."

- ROBERT LOUIS STEVENSON

Ask any new personal trainer about his or her biggest challenge, and it's likely to be selling. Few trainers start out knowing how to sell, let alone sell effectively. But once you understand what selling really is, and how to go about it, I promise you'll feel more confident—and more importantly, make more sales.

The Art of Selling

At its heart, selling consists of two things: understanding your potential clients and making your skill set meaningful to them. If you can do that, they will want to work with you, and nobody else.

w trainer, you have to be able to market the skills you have.
experience, you also market the results that you've helped
your clients achieve. So, the first step is to identify what sets you apart
from other trainers, which you learned about last chapter. You need to
know why you're a better choice than the competition, and to highlight
that for potential clients.

Complete this sentence: *I differ from other trainers in that:* _____.
List at least three attributes that make you special. Have you received
training to work with specific groups of clients? Have you lost fifty
pounds and kept it off through lifestyle changes? Are you knowledgeable about a particular medical condition?

Then think about the benefits you can provide clients. Be as detailed
and thorough as possible, and don't worry about whether those benefits are unique to you as a trainer. For example, you can help clients lose
weight, become more toned, add muscle, and perform better at sports.
The more benefits you can explain to a potential client, the more likely
a client will respond to one or more of those benefits.

I keep a handout posted in my office that reads:

Why Use a Personal Trainer?

- *Optimize your workout time*
- *Ensure proper form*
- *Accurate assessment*
- *Exercise safety through proper form and adequate rest*
- *Accountability*
- *Everybody benefits from a trainer. The top athletes in the world still use trainers so "knowing enough" to work out on your own is not an excuse.*
- *A trainer will push you beyond your comfort zone while staying within your limits. You won't push yourself beyond your comfort zone.*
- *Personalization*

- *Motivation*
- *Niche specialties*
  - o *Cardiac rehab*
  - o *Older adults*
  - o *Post-rehab for an injury*
  - o *Body fat loss*
  - o *Muscle gain*
  - o *Improve athletic performance*
  - o *Chronic illness (training with Parkinson's etc.)*
  - o *Pre/post natal training*
  - o *Post-menopausal training (staving off osteoporosis)*
- *Improve flexibility with assisted stretching*
- *Easy access to a community and support system*

I give potential clients a copy of this list so they can see the benefits of training and what I can help them with in black and white. I suggest you create your own handout to share with potential clients. The more reasons you can give people to hire you, the more likely they are to do so.

Communicating your Value

I started working at Body + Soul wanting nothing to do with the business end of training. Like many trainers, all I wanted to do was train clients. I figured that an appointed salesperson would handle the business aspect and I would stick to what I did best. Fortunately I quickly realized that sales are integral to being a successful personal trainer, and that selling doesn't mean tricking someone into buying an overpriced product. Selling means getting a client to want to work with me—in other words, *I* am the product!

I was selling myself, and I wasn't overpriced. I knew I offered value. Selling consisted of educating the client on that value. That didn't mean I was effective at the beginning. As a new trainer, I bombarded a potential client with everything that I knew about the body and training.

Fortunately, one of my mentors explained that I was working too hard to try and impress clients, and suggested instead that I focus on educating clients about what *specifically* I could help them with. That's how you communicate your value.

But before you can convince a client of your value, you must gather as much information as possible about him or her. Find out about past struggles, injuries, goals, and issues, and tailor your services specifically toward that client.

If the client has an issue or injury that you've dealt with before, tell him about your experience with his issue and how you've helped somebody with a similar problem. If the client has an issue that you don't know a lot about, I recommend you research the condition and send him information about it to show that you'll go the "extra 10 percent as a trainer. (Don't tell him you'll send reading material—surprise him. It's more memorable.)

Clients increasingly want to train with somebody who knows about their specific issues, and by highlighting your unique qualifications (e.g., experience helping increase bone density in post-menopausal women), you may attract clients who otherwise would be reluctant to walk through your door.

Keep in mind that after you've established your reputation as a trainer, communicating your value becomes less important. Once you've successfully worked with a number of clients, they'll go out of their way to tell friends about you. At that point, new clients will already be aware of your value and closing the sale becomes much easier.

TRAINING TIP:

Understand your clients and the role you play in their lives. Educate them about your value using specific examples and describe how you can help them.

The 5-Step Selling Process

What's the first thing a potential client says to you in a sales meeting? It's probably something like:

- "How much does it cost?"
- "How often do I need to see you?"
- "How can I start?"

Your first reaction may be to answer the question, but I suggest that you instead use this simple five-step process to close sales.

Step 1: Ask, "What is it you want to achieve?"
The potential client has already invested time in speaking with you. Now it's time for you to prove your worth, and asking this question right away shifts both control and focus. You have placed yourself in the driver's seat by asking the client to tell you about himself. Listen to what the person tells you and take careful notes. Ask if there is a specific reason why he is coming to you, and try to determine what will create an emotional connection for your client. [I'll talk more about how to do this in chapter 6.] Once you know what the client wants to achieve, you can sketch out a path for him.

It's important during these initial meetings to be quiet and let the client speak. Often, all that I'll do is ask questions and paraphrase their answers. Make sure you ask every potential client the following questions:

- Any injuries?
- What are your goals?
- Have you been a member of a gym before?
- Have you had a trainer before?
- Why did you quit (or not achieve success) previously?
- What are your expectations of me?

Remember to be quiet and let the client speak after each question. Pause for several seconds when you think the person is finished before you begin talking.

Step 2: Sell results, not packages.

Once you know what the client hopes to achieve, hammer out a plan for your client that will meet his goals. If you think that his goals will take 4 workouts a week then give a brief description of why and what each workout will entail. Depending on the client, you may decide to give an overview on the physiology of adaptation and what they can expect. (I like to describe cross-bridge formation, DOMS (delayed onset muscle soreness), and the difference between neural and muscular gains to show that I'm research-focused and don't just count repetitions.

Some clients appreciate a more detailed description while others do not. Gauge your client's reaction to your plan and the reasons for it to determine whether you should go into more detail. You might ask something like, "Do you want to know a little about how soreness works and why it is not a great indicator of how hard you worked?" Let the client lead you in terms of how much detail you provide.

Step 3: Address objections.

If your client has objections or questions, address them now. Say something like, "What do you think about the plan?" and then listen to what he says.

It's rare to make a sale without dealing with objections. Getting a trainer is a big decision and clients want to make sure that you're worth the bread in addition to being the right choice for *them.*

I recommend not bringing up the cost of training before the client has been sold on what you have to offer. A rate of, say, $50/hour will be too expensive if the client doesn't understand your value. Before you talk money, a client should have spoken to you at length about his exercise goals, history, previous challenges, injuries, and any possible training interruptions coming up. In addition, clients should be aware of your credentials, specializations (if they apply to them), the frequency they need to train, and the general overall plan for the workouts, even if that's subject to change. In short, they should be pumped to train and convinced that you're the right person to get them the results they want. Then your value is understood and cost becomes less of a problem.

If a potential client asks what you charge before you talk about your value, I suggest gently changing the subject. If the person still demands to know the cost, tell him, but your chances of making the sale go way down at that point. (Those clients will likely end up at the cheapest facility and there isn't much that you can do.)

Address any reservations or concerns about hiring a trainer your client may have. No matter what the objection, I use the following technique as a simple guideline:

1. Paraphrase the question and repeat it back in the form of a statement. This shows the client that you understand and are listening.
2. Depending on the objection, you may need to re-educate her on the value that you bring to the table. Demonstrate why you're the person who can help her because you have the skills to address her specific problem(s).
3. If a potential client says, "I need to think about it," ask what it is she needs to think about. There's always a tangible reason behind this excuse.

Here are some common objections or issues clients have and how to address them:

- **Lack of time.** If a potential client lacks time to train, discuss different types of workout routines suited to her goals that will work within her timeline. For example, if you have a client who wants to lose fat, discuss metabolic workouts and how much more "bang for your buck" these workouts will get your client as opposed to steady-state cardio.

- **A previous injury.** Make sure you understand the injury. I keep a database on the most common injuries I come across. (When I come across a new injury, I make sure to add it to the database.) Contained within that database are papers varying in complexity describing the injury and rehabilitation protocols. If I'm familiar with the injury, I proceed to pummel the client with knowledge, so to speak. If I'm not familiar with the injury, I use the line "I can help you with that." Either way, I print out some information for the client on the spot and hand it to her. That shows again that I'm willing to go the extra 10 percent.

- **A previous bad experience with a trainer.** Don't bad-mouth anybody. Always give a former trainer the benefit of the doubt, but educate the client as to how you would treat the situation differently. Say the client didn't feel the previous trainer listened to her; I would tell her I was sorry about that but that as a client, she can call me during the day or email me any time. I also remind her that during our sessions (or anytime she sees me in the gym—as long as I'm not with a client!), she's welcome to speak about anything. Whatever the bad experience was, show that you're going to deal with it differently.

- **A know-it-all attitude.** A fair number of clients believe they don't need a trainer because they "know what they're doing." When I hear something like this, I get a thorough understanding of a client's previous and current workouts and goals. I will then highlight several points where she can improve, and if I can, I provide the person with research on whatever her goals are (like hypertrophy, fat loss, or toning). While this person may not hire you immediately, I suggest you stay in contact with this person. She may wind up approaching you and asking you to train her.

- **Cost.** Cost is a different type of obstacle. If you have demonstrated your value to a potential client, cost should not even be an obstacle! Yes, some people can't afford a trainer, but the fact that you're a little cheaper or more expensive than another trainer shouldn't matter. If $80/hour is too expensive, so is $70. But if a client understands your value, she won't balk at $80/hour versus $70/hour. Other than setting up payment plans when necessary, I'm against negotiating the price of training. It's important to stick to your value, but you can be creative in making a plan that will work for a client who can't train with you as often. (I'll give you some examples later in this chapter.)

Step 4: Get the buy-in.

Before bringing up price you should book the person into your schedule according to the plan you've sketched out. Having clients commit to training times and dates makes it harder for them to balk at the sale. Then, you can discuss money.

I suggest you have a professional sales sheet that details the different packages you offer. Then you can offer clients two options (the best and second best), citing their goals. I might say something like, "Sally, you mentioned that you really want to give this your all and we've set some pretty lofty but attainable goals of X, Y, and Z. In order to hit these goals by the date you mentioned, I'm going to need you training with me 3x/week and twice on your own, where I'll give you a full plan of what to do. The most cost-effective option is the 50-pack of sessions and it will take our training over 3 months to finish. This is more than enough time to get measurable results. If that's too big of a commitment for you off the bat, we also offer a 20-session package. Please also remember that our sessions are fully refundable so you don't need to be worried about getting stuck with a larger package if something happens."

I like to give two options because it makes for a softer sell, and gives the client a choice. I also remind the client that she can get a refund if she decides not to pursue training with me.

Step 5: Get creative if necessary.

You won't always need to use step 5, but you will have clients that can't train with you as often as your plan requires. That's when you get creative to help your clients reach their goals.

For example, instead of giving a client a workout each time she comes in, you might give her an hour-long lesson in the weight room so that she is comfortable working out once or twice a week on her own. Or you might not even be in the weight room! I've taken clients into our conference room to go over their workout plans. The idea is to provide your clients with the tools they need to train on their own, if necessary.

If your client can't work out with you as often as you'd like, tell her what she'll be responsible for on her own, and get her to buy into it. Remember how to manipulate price. This may involve creativity on your part to make the sale but be careful not to prejudge a client and always start high. If the client's goals require her to work out 5 times a week, be honest and educate her about why this is so. I'm always surprised at how often a client will offer to train with me more frequently when I properly communicate what she needs to do to achieve her goals.

For example, Vlad was a member of the gym who would often ask me questions but he never asked to train with me. I always answered his questions, and was surprised when he finally asked me to be his personal trainer.

Vlad was recovering from rotator cuff surgery and didn't have much money. Having completed physiotherapy, he wanted an exercise routine that he could do 3 times/week with a focus on continual strengthening of the shoulder and functional strength. He couldn't afford to work with me this often, but wanted a program that constantly changed to keep him interested but still focused on his problem shoulder.

After educating Vlad on the necessity of progression, we agreed to meet once a week for 7 weeks. Vlad's form was already pretty good, and I was confident that I could show Vlad a movement and he would be able to emulate it the following week. He also knew that he could contact me with any questions. I devised a workout plan for him that included 7 categories:

- Pull;
- Push;
- Mid-back/shoulder stability;
- Core stability/anti-rotation;
- Core rotation/flexion;
- Legs (hip dominant);
- Legs (quad dominant); and
- Arms.

I included 4 or 5 exercises in each group and instructed Vlad to choose 1-2 exercises from each category per workout, focusing on shoulder stability and core strength. Our sessions consisted of making Vlad comfortable with the given exercises, and to make sure that he knew when the weight was appropriate and when it needed to be increased.

When we were done, Vlad had the freedom to choose from a large assortment of workouts. The exercises I included were specific to his needs and he knew how to progress. I gave Vlad the freedom and knowledge to make his own workouts within certain parameters, and he got much more value from this plan—yet he was still able to afford it.

TRAINING TIP:

Be creative. If a client has financial constraints, find a solution that will work for him and help him reach his goals.

With another client, Lisa, I had to overcome the negative experiences she'd had with other trainers. When I asked her about her history, I learned that she'd always trained using low weights in a circuit. She'd been told that it was the best way to fat burn since her heart rate would be up the whole workout. Second, none of her previous trainers had given her detailed instruction, so Lisa was clueless about how to work out on her own. She'd meet with her trainer once or twice a week, and then tried to work out on her own, but she hadn't achieved the results she wanted.

I developed a plan for Lisa that would enable her to meet her goals. Her initial goal was to lose 25 pounds, but I wanted her to put on muscle and get stronger. I educated Lisa on the difference between absolute weight and body composition, and told her that if she was going to train with me, she was going to train like a power lifter. I explained that the added muscle would increase her BMR (basal metabolic rate) and that the workouts would have a greater TEE (Thermic Effect of Exercise). The stubborn weight would come off as a by-product.

In addition, I told Lisa that I didn't want to see her every week. I was going to force her to be self-sufficient. I therefore proposed an arrangement to Lisa where we would meet 3 times in one week. This would enable me to teach her enough to feel comfortable for the next month. I wanted to make sure she never left another gym feeling disoriented again! I was always available for questions, so she knew from the minute she walked into the gym she knew what she had to accomplish and had already acquired the requisite self-efficacy to complete the task.

I gave Lisa a power workout that contained fewer exercises for her to master. In short, I wanted Lisa to feel great doing 8 exercises in a workout as opposed to feeling confused trying to master 20+ exercises. So what happened?

In her first year, she got unbelievable results. She reached her goal of losing the 25 pounds while eating more than ever (I did get her to keep a diary and worked with her on making proper choices). She's also incredibly strong, and most of all, Lisa is a much more confident person in and out of the gym.

All it took with Lisa was a minor push in the right direction. I listened carefully to what didn't work and made sure not to repeat the mistakes. I then devised a program that was completely different, that she could afford, and that I knew she could master. By helping Lisa become confident and knowledgeable in the gym, I gained a lifetime client.

I shared these stories to remind you that no two clients are the same. Often it takes a little creativity to sell clients on training and retain them. While it would be great if every client wanted to train with you 3 times a week for life, that's not realistic!

TRAINING TIP:

Educate and empower your clients. You can create a client army that will go out of their way to spread the word about how amazing you are. That's the key to being a career trainer.

Inside Info – Marc Lebert

Marc Lebert is the inventor of the Lebert Equalizer and owner of Fitness NATION.

Like many others, his formal education is not in fitness or health sciences. He first completed a degree in law and security and then went back to school to study psychology. When he graduated, his job at a squash/fitness club included cleaning the pool, folding towels, signing up members, and training clients. When the club was bought out, Marc decided to leave and has been working for himself for the last 15 years.

Marc's business is almost solely based on group exercise He markets through word of mouth and referral incentives, and travels to numerous trade shows yearly to show off the Lebert Equalizer

Marc's 3 keys to succeeding as a personal trainer are:

1. Personality – Never forget to have fun

2. Compassion – Listen but don't fall into clients "loops or patterns". Learn how to spot when they repeat behaviours, language, and internal dialogue that are self limiting and unconscious. Have compassion for where they are and lead them into new patterns of thinking, and eventually their behaviours will match their goals.

3. Passion – You can't make someone love fitness, but you can love it yourself and that may rub off on your clients.

Marc's words to live by:

"Do your best to lose your clients by giving them everything you have. They will never leave. Life begins just outside your comfort zone – do some public speaking, a few extra reps and get out there!"

Marc Lebert is the owner of Fitness NATION and the creator of the Lebert Equalizer. His website is www.lebertfitness.com

Selling in Action

Not every sale takes place on the gym floor. I'd like to share an example of how you can find clients anywhere—if you know how to sell to them.

Several years ago at a party, I met Jeff, who suffered from chronic pain. It appeared that he'd been injured working with a personal trainer months before. Jeff hadn't gone back to the gym after that, but because he worked in construction, he'd been forced to constantly medicate himself. I asked Jeff about what had happened since then, and he told me that he'd quit working with the trainer and had tried acupuncture and massage therapy on a weekly basis but that the pain always returned. In addition, Jeff wasn't able to go mountain biking and was afraid to drive his motorcycle. His quality of life was severely compromised.

Normally I would take notes while talking with a potential client, but since I was at a party I didn't have that luxury. I already had valuable information that I could use to make a sale, though:

- He couldn't do activities that he loved such as mountain biking and riding his motorcycle.
- He'd had a motorcycle accident in the past, which left him with permanent shoulder and knee damage in addition to his lower back pain.
- He was well-educated and appreciated well-researched health and fitness information.
- His view of trainers had been tarnished as he viewed his previous trainer as being responsible for his injury. In addition, that trainer didn't follow proper programming and Jeff never saw any results.
- Jeff didn't want to pay any more money for acupuncture or massage therapy because it only helped the symptoms, not the underlying problem. He wanted to address the problem and get back into shape.

Keeping these factors in mind, I spoke to Jeff about his previous experience. I made sure to avoid criticizing the trainer but highlighted the importance of proper exercise choice and progression. We talked about the importance of a building from the bottom up and having a full dynamic warm-up and mobility work to prepare for exercises like the deadlift, and how the glutes and abs must be activated properly to avoid injury. We also talked about the benefits and limitations of disciplines such as acupuncture and massage. In combination with a proper exercise program, they can be effective treatments, but they won't create proper movement patterns or develop muscle. Finally, we talked about how he would feel when he would be pain-free and could get back to activities that he loves. I wanted to make our conversation emotional for him.

I couldn't give him a timeline because he had not completed an assessment, and I needed more information about his shoulder and knee issues before I created a plan for him. At the end of the conversation, I gave him my card and told him to contact me if he wanted any more information, and asked him for his email address. At no point did I ask him to train with me or even mention the gym I worked at. When I got home that night, I forwarded him a review article on lower back rehabilitation and told him to call if he had any questions about the article. (Note that I never mentioned during our conversation that I would send him any info. I made a note in my phone to send the study to him when I got home.) It was the extra effort that refreshed his mind about our conversation the following day and showed him that I was a different breed of trainer willing to go the extra 10 percent.

Three days later, Jeff called to make an appointment to train with me. Without selling, I had a committed client. The cost of the training sessions didn't matter because he understood the value. When clients understand your value, they'll be happy to pay whatever you charge. On the other hand, if clients aren't sold on your value, you could be the cheapest trainer in the world and still be too expensive.

I wouldn't have said that I could have helped him with his back pain if I wasn't qualified to do so. After a complete assessment (and getting medical clearance), we started a glutes activation plan that included showing him how to stand, sit, and carry objects properly to reduce pain. Within five months, he was pain-free and stronger than he'd ever been—and I had another committed client who spreads the word about what I do.

Without one word concerning sales, I was able to take a client whose view of trainers had been seriously tarnished and I converted him into a great client and an inspiring story! Since then, he's written a great testimonial that I use to sell myself to other clients who suffer from lower back pain.

TRAINING TIP:

Listening is more important than talking. Make sure you know what your client's problems and goals are, and demonstrate how you can help. A client (especially one who's had a prior bad experience) will notice that you're different right from the start.

POINTS TO REMEMBER:

- The ability to sell yourself and your value to potential clients is an essential aspect of succeeding as a trainer.

- The more you know about a potential client, the more easily you can sell to that person.

- Selling doesn't come easy to most trainers. It's a skill that needs to be learned the same way that squat progressions are, but you will get better with time.

Chapter 5

One on One: Developing Client Relationships

"The creation of a thousand forests is in one acorn."

- RALPH WALDO EMERSON

Your relationship with your client starts the first time you interact with that person. Maybe you greeted her at the gym. Maybe you had a brief conversation with him in the weight room. Or maybe your first conversation was when he approached you about hiring you to train him.

But once a client hires you, your trainer/client relationship officially begins. Create a strong bond from the start, and you'll not only help your clients achieve their goals—you'll find that happy clients are more than willing to recommend you and refer friends, family members, and colleagues to you.

You probably already know that it takes much more time to sign a new client or customer than to retain a current one. So keep this fact in mind: *The work to build a strong bond with a client pales in comparison to the work involved in continually attracting and signing new clients.*

Breaking the Ice

Developing great relationships with a client starts with getting to know them on a personal level, but most clients seem reluctant to open up early on. So how do you quickly break down the barriers a client puts up?

First, listen. You learned last chapter that it's important to listen to a potential client during the selling process. Now that you're training your client, it's even more important. Ask your client how he's feeling, or how his day has been. Small talk can help break the ice as you start a training session. Often clients are anxious or feel awkward; they're not trying to be rude. Don't take it personally. As your client gets to know you better, chances are good that he or she will become more open with you.

I find that clients let down some of their barriers when I tell a semi-embarrassing or funny story about my own life. It eases the tension and shows that I'm human. I recommend keeping a couple of stories in reserve at all times. The best stories are those that relate to the gym (for example, being unable to press a too-heavy weight at the bottom of a bench press, and calling somebody else to lift the bar off of you).

Sharing this kind of personal experience reminds clients that everybody struggles with exercise and they shouldn't be afraid to fail. In fact, they should embrace failure. (Later, when I discuss the physiology of skill acquisition, you will understand why "failing with purpose" is imperative to your client's success.)

One of my favourite stories to use is to describe my first experience curling. The short version is that I found I lacked curling skills. In fact, the first time I tried it, I fell on the ice, bruised my hip, and walked with a limp for two weeks! This story shows clients that personal trainers struggle with new exercise endeavours too. Reminding clients of that can help reduce anxiety.

As a trainer, pay attention not only to your client's words but body language and actions as well. You can learn a lot about someone's personality and comfort level just by watching how she interacts with you and with other people. As you get to know your client better, you'll be better able to figure out what will motivate and inspire her [you'll learn more about that in chapter 8] but at the outset, you want to create a relationship of trust. To help create a great relationship early, I suggest these techniques:

- Smile. To paraphrase Dale Carnegie, a smile lets clients know you're happy to see them.
- Make eye contact. That lets clients know you're interested in what they have to say, and that they're important to you.
- Use isopraxism, or mimicking behaviour. This nonverbal and usually subconscious behaviour helps establish rapport and empathy. It means you follow your client's lead; if she speaks softly, so do you. If he laughs, you laugh as well.
- Stay on their level. Body positioning is important. For example, if your client is sitting on a bench and you want to speak to her, get on her level by crouching next to her. Never "talk down" to a client.

5 Simple Ways to Create Client Relationships

Want to build loyal, lasting relationships with clients? Use these five strategies:

#1: Educate them.
Most of your clients will come to you knowing little about fitness. Indoctrinate them into the workout culture. Teach them the

jargon. Tell them what words like set, rep, hypertrophy, and even RDL (short for Romanian deadlift) mean. Make sure that they know why they're doing the primary exercises and what energy system they're developing.

Smart clients are confident clients, and they'll jump at the opportunity to tell their friends and family that they performed 2 sets of 8 reps of the deadlift—which was aptly named because it was developed in ancient Rome to lift the dead off of the battlefield.

Educated clients also feel more part of the gym. Retention will increase, and your clients will be less likely to "relapse" back into inactivity.

#2: Welcome them.

Make your clients part of the gym community. Introduce them to all of the staff and their fellow members; they should be the most popular people in the gym. When they feel comfortable, they're likely to chat other members up—and guess what they'll be talking about? Their great trainer!

Clients who feel welcome in the gym stay longer, plain and simple. The gym becomes a place not only to work out, but also a place to socialize and have fun. And the longer they're in the gym, the more likely they are to become part of your "client army" and spread the word about you to anyone who will listen. They may even go out of their way to bring in friends and family not just because they enjoy the gym, but also because they want to show off their popularity.

TRAINING TIP:

Build your army by making your clients popular. They will chat up new members for you, stay longer, and bring more people into the club.

Strategy #3: Surprise them.

You probably already know that you should "touch" your clients regularly by sending thoughtful emails such as restaurant recommendations or new studies they may be interested in. This is a great idea, but you'll make a bigger impression if you don't mention it in advance.

When I'm training someone and get the idea to send a client a relevant article, for example, I make a note on my clipboard and continue the workout. The next day, I send the email, saying something like, "I thought you would enjoy this—it's what we were speaking about yesterday."

That makes a bigger impact than telling your client you'll send her something and then keeping your word. The surprise effect keeps you in your clients' minds even during off days and shows that you think of them outside of training hours. (You know you're developing a good relationship when clients send *you* funny jokes, restaurant advice, or relevant articles on *their* off days!)

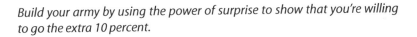

TRAINING TIP:

Build your army by using the power of surprise to show that you're willing to go the extra 10 percent.

Strategy #4: Celebrate them.

Each month, I give one client an award that I've developed. The award is given to a client who has gone above and beyond, training-wise. I give the person a badge with his name on it that he can keep, and profile him on my website, highlighting his accomplishments.

I highly recommend you develop a similar award for your clients. I've found that since I started the monthly badge, my clients work harder and cancel fewer workouts. They all want to win! The result? They all reach their goals faster.

The award also brings my clients together and creates a sense of community and healthy competition among them. I've found that clients show off their badges, and email their friends about their write-ups, which means more exposure for me as they reach their goals. Giving out well-deserved awards can be win/win for you as a trainer.

Strategy #5: Empower them.

When you do a great job, your clients will want to spread the word about their results—and about you. Make it easy for them by always having business cards on hand, and make sure your clients always have them, too.

You should also have something in writing—say, a brief bio and a description of the services that you offer. Include client testimonials and any specialties, and offer it to clients. You should also have your brochure or pamphlet available for download on your (and your company's) website.

TRAINING TIP:

Make it easy for your clients to pass on info about you to their contacts.

Handling Prior Negative Experiences

In the coming chapters you'll learn about getting your clients excited about working out and about exercise programming and progression. But let me address an important issue here—what to do when a client has had a bad experience with a trainer in the past.

It may have been that the trainer's style just didn't work for the client, that the trainer didn't give the client enough attention, that the client was injured, or that the trainer simply didn't listen to the client. Regardless, make sure that you know what happened before, and don't repeat it! Communicate that to your client. You might say something like, "What happened before was the past, and we can't change that. What we can change, though, is the future. So let's focus our energy on your journey moving forward." Or, you might say, "I understand that you don't feel like your previous trainer listened to you. Well, the more information that I know about you the better, so please do not hold anything back! My clients will tell you that one of the reasons they train with me is because I pay close attention to them, and I assure you that you'll find this to be true."

Often a client may have felt ignored or taken for granted by a trainer. If you suspect this is the case, show the person you're different. Surprise them with an email, or go the "extra 10 percent" with a handout that shows you've been thinking about them.

> **TRAINING TIP:**
>
> *Make sure clients know that you're different, and that you won't repeat any problems they had with trainers in the past.*

Inside Info – Scott Tate

Scott Tate is a personal trainer in Toronto specializing in chronic disease clients, specifically fibromyaligia, chronic lyme disease, and Parkinson's. He also heads up the continuing education department for a multi-gym company in Toronto.

Scott began his career by volunteering in physiotherapy clinics throughout high school and university. Helping friends in the gym and in sport led him to a job at the University of Guelph's Athletic Center in Ontario, Canada. After finishing his Human Kinetics degree, Scott stayed on at university to study Applied Human Nutrition. He left after two years to embark on a career in personal training.

He has worked in boutique-style training facilities and trained clients in-home. He started a company with the sole purpose of connecting practitioners to provide well-rounded inter-professional care. When Scott realized he needed more space and better focused attention from his clients, he moved to a boutique training gym in Toronto. His business is referral-based through clients that he's already helped and other health-care practitioners he's connected with.

Scott's 3 keys to succeeding as a personal trainer are:

1. Be passionate about helping people – If you don't care, neither will they. If you're in this only for the paycheck it will show. Passion rubs off. Potential clients can sense it and will immediately be drawn to you while existing clients will never want to leave.

2. Have patience and empathy – We never truly know what's going on in our clients lives. Stressors beyond our control get in the way of their workouts. If you want to help your clients patience and empathy goes a long way.

3. Know that neither you, nor any system, is perfect – Continually improve. Strive to get better and never be satisfied. Preventative medicine is still young but it's the most powerful drug ever designed. Keeping up to date with methods will ensure you stay on top.

Scott's words to live by:

"Are you in this to help people or to help your bank? If it's the people that pump you up, the bank will do its thing. If it's dollars that drive you, take another route."

Scott Tate is a personal trainer and kinesiologist. He currently sits on the board for the Ontario Kinesiology Association and is the continuing education coach for Body + Soul Fitness. He can be reached at Scott@bodyandsoul.ca

Every Client Counts

I'd like to share an example of how strong client relationships pay off, not only for them (they reach their goals!) but for you as a trainer, too. I started training Cindy years ago. Cindy was in her 60s and suffered from shoulder and knee pain and wanted to lose some weight. While she'd tried numerous exercise programs, she had no gym experience.

I initially focused on creating a comfortable gym environment for Cindy, and within a few months, she was already feeling stronger and fitter. She referred her friend Pam to me. Like Cindy, Pam too had no gym experience and was apprehensive about working with a trainer. They asked if they could train together, and I agreed. I educated them about what we were doing, introduced them to other gym members, and kept in touch with them when they weren't in the gym.

They both had their share of aches, pains, and doubts, but they stuck with the program and started to progress. Within weeks, they were noticing how much stronger they were, not only at the gym but at home as well. Pam was glowing when she walked into the gym one day, and announced that she had climbed up on a ladder—something she hadn't done in years. And Cindy, who'd had some mobility issues, stood up one day without holding onto anything, and didn't even realize it until she was already up! These accomplishments (what I call "aha!" moments, which I'll talk about next chapter) kept them motivated.

Today Pam and Cindy are strong, fit, and healthy, and have become members of my client army. Both continually send friends and colleagues to me. (At one point, about two-thirds of my clients were direct referrals from either Pam or Cindy! That's how much of an impact they had on my success.)

But here's my point. Personal training success goes outside the boundaries of technical knowledge. Lots of qualified trainers could have helped them get in better shape. But I was unique because I made the experience *comfortable* for them. Because of that, they both achieved goals they thought were beyond them. And they now look forward to the gym!

Keeping in Touch

You spend just a few hours out of the week with any client, so staying in touch through methods other than face-to-face is important. At the moment, I manage 6 email accounts, 2 Facebook accounts, 2 phone lines, and I use Twitter and text messaging as well. I personally answer all messages from clients, friends, colleagues, readers of the PTDC, and media/advertising inquires. It's a lot to keep track of, and I'm currently consolidating how I connect with clients.

Your clients will dictate how you keep in touch, but you should always be easy to reach. Here's how I stay in contact:

- **Text messaging.** Text messaging is by far the most common way I keep in touch with my clients. Text messages are quick, easy, and garner fast responses.
- **Email.** Email plays a similar role for me; I use it when I have a longer message to send to a client, or to pass along relevant arti-cles a client may be interested in.
- **Phone.** The phone is the best way to truly connect with your client and the best way for consulting with a potential client. Unless you're scheduling an appointment, the phone should be your communication method of choice as it's more immediate and gives you a chance to ask about how a client's day is going. When a client gives you a potential referral, get that person on the phone as quick as possible and start compiling all of the informa-tion you need to make the sale. The window of opportunity might be small if you don't build the relationship immediately.

What about Social Media?

Social media is one of the most efficient and effective ways to keep in touch with clients; here's a brief overview of how you can use it to your advantage:

- **Facebook**. I hold both personal and public Facebook accounts; the personal account is limited to my close friends and family. However, I have about 2,500 friends on my public account who represent a cross-section of clients, colleagues, and trainers from throughout the world. My public account has been a great place not only to interact with my current clients but also to generate referrals. When a client reaches a goal, I congratulate him on Facebook and "tag" him in the post so it shows up on his wall. When I run group classes, I take photos and post them on Facebook, tagging each participant congratulating them on their efforts. Facebook is a great community-builder for clients and an easy way to keep up with their birthdays and other special events.

- **LinkedIn**. Most of my clients are professionals and almost all of them have LinkedIn accounts. I created my own account, added my clients, and asked some of them for recommendations. LinkedIn takes little or no maintenance; it's a place where potential clients can get a quick snapshot of you and read testimonials. If you don't have a website yet, LinkedIn should be your calling card.

- **Twitter**. I use Twitter for professionally networking but haven't found it useful for connecting with clients. Only 3 of my clients follow me. I do however mention those three in tweets when I can.

- **Blogging**. If you have time to create and maintain a blog, it can help you get your message out and stay connected with clients. You can set up a blog and host it for free on sites like wordpress.com. Your blog can be a calling card for you, and let you go the extra 10 percent for clients. You can post your favourite recipe, write about new research, or provide instructions on completing a difficult exercise, for example. Blogging can also be a fun way to express yourself, but keep your posts positive and on point. Rants won't do you any good.

Respecting Client/Trainer Boundaries

In a field like personal training, where you work in close physical proximity, it's important that you understand the importance of setting appropriate boundaries. First, I advise you to use your intuition. If you feel uncomfortable with a client, address the situation right away.

Always avoid sexual innuendo or other comments that could be misconstrued by a client. If a *client* uses innuendo during a workout or otherwise makes you uncomfortable, pointedly ignore it the first time. Often the client will feel awkward and refrain in the future. If a client persists in making lewd or inappropriate comments, however, ask the person to stop. If the behaviour continues, speak to your manager (if you have one) and ask to have the client reassigned. If you work for yourself, you may simply have to "fire" your client. No client is worth risking your reputation.

While a lot of clients (including me) use text messaging as the method of choice to communicate with clients, it should be used with care. Text messages should be kept professional and to the point; I only use them to quickly confirm a session or schedule a session. If a client texts you at odd hours (such as late at night), I suggest you respond during regular business hours or send an email in reply. It's a subtle way of training your client to respect your privacy. Or call the client instead.

Then there's Facebook. Clients will want to be your friends on Facebook, so you can either make yourself unsearchable (controlling who sees your profile), or you can set up two accounts, a public one with your real name and a private profile with an assumed name. Your public profile should be kept *very* professional. Monitor what people write on your wall and remove anything controversial, keep your status updates appropriate, and remember that employers often look at Facebook accounts as part of the hiring process.

There's nothing wrong with grabbing a quick bite to eat with a client after a workout or meeting over a cup of coffee for a change of scenery. This can strengthen your relationship with a client, but I suggest you avoid encounters that could appear inappropriate, like having dinner alone with a member of the opposite sex. If you're invited, just say "no" or ask permission to bring your significant other. That should send the right message to your client.

What if…

So, what if you have feelings for a client that you want to act on? Stop training the person immediately. Pursuing a romantic relationship with a client is a sticky subject and could potentially have legal ramifications, so always err on the side of caution.

TRAINING TIP:

Understand the professional relationship that exists between you and your client, and make sure that you don't send the wrong message to your client (or anyone else) by your behaviour.

POINTS TO REMEMBER:

- It takes less time to create lasting relationships with current clients than to constantly look for new clients.

- Make your clients feel comfortable and popular at the gym, and they will work out more frequently and reach their goals.

- Keep in touch with your clients, even when they're not at the gym. This will help cement relationships.

Chapter 6

Ignition with the Excitation System

"Let's not forget that the little emotions are the great captains of our lives and we obey them without realizing it."

- VINCENT VAN GOGH

As you learned from the story I shared last chapter, your job as a trainer goes beyond simply developing training regimes or teaching clients moves. Successful personal trainers not only have passion for what they do, they're able to incite passion in the clients as well. I believe your real job as a trainer is to create an emotional connection with exercise for your clients so that they will look forward to working out and stay with it for life. You do that by creating what I call "aha!" moments with clients.

My First Aha! Moment

I started getting serious about lifting weights in high school but struggled early on. I didn't have any mentors and I really didn't know what I was doing. I was close to quitting when I started dating my high school sweetheart. I was young, inexperienced and self-conscious, but I remember when my girlfriend was impressed with my body. She was surprised I had some muscle on me! Apparently that year of working out had made a difference, and I remember how confident and proud I felt.

That was my first "aha!" moment and it was a powerful one. From that moment I was hooked, and I've never thought about leaving the gym since.

TRAINING TIP:

When you train clients, remember your "aha!" moment(s)—and strive to create those for them as soon as possible.

The Excitation System

Once I understood the importance of creating "aha!" moments for clients, I developed the Excitation System. This system helps create enthusiasm and develop motivation in the clients you work with. In order to sell a client on a workout, you must get her excited. Light that fire so that nothing will get in the way of her progress. When I introduce a workout to a client, I use the following 5-step process:

- Paraphrase her goals. I remind the client of her goals and encourage her to visualize herself meeting them.
- Give a brief overview of the workout. I explain that what we're doing is the best option for the client.

- Go over the primary exercises. I'll describe the movement, and may show the client a video of someone performing it properly. If I'm introducing the workout for the first time, I'll explain the importance of the primary exercises and that their progression will be based on these exercises.
- Address any potential limitations. When a client has an injury or imbalance or has a break in training coming up, I'll talk about how we'll address each issue.
- Remind about proper warm-up and "prehab," or injury prevention. This will help keep your client healthy and injury-free.

The 10 to 15 minutes it takes you to use the Excitation System will save you hours later on. The system reinforces clients' goals, gives them a chance to ask questions, helps them understand progression and how we'll monitor it, addresses any barriers, and educates the client on the importance of warm-up and prehab exercises.

You won't be able to get a single client continual results unless you have her full commitment. Your job is to be a facilitator; you cannot work out for your client. I promise that the client won't give 100 percent if she doesn't understand or buy into the program you're giving her. If you have a client that you think isn't giving it her all, I suggest that you sit down and run her through the excitation questions. You'll be surprised at what a short candid conversation can do for her motivation. Once you finish the talk and get on the floor, your client will be raring to go!

Using the Excitation System

Now that you know what the Excitation system is, let's take a look at how to use it with a client. My client, Jenny, was 36 and a long-time runner who wanted to run faster and add some muscle; she originally had some muscle imbalances and inflexibility we'd addressed during the anatomical adaptation phase. Now I wanted her to start performing heavier lifting. After welcoming her to my office, and reviewing her progress so far, we had the following conversation:

Jon: Jenny, I'm really happy with the gains that you've made these past 6 weeks. Already you're moving a lot better! In fact, you're now ready to progress onto more challenging workouts. Do you remember our initial assessment? I told you that I wanted you to train for power after the initial anatomical adaptation phase. This is because power training will help you push off faster with you running in addition to helping you build nice dense muscle.

Jenny: I remember. So what's next?

Jon: I've chosen two exercises for you specific to your body type and goals. They are the clean and press and Romanian deadlift.

Jenny: Deadlift?

Jon: Don't be put off by the name! The deadlift is an incredibly effective exercise for strengthening the posterior chain, the connection between the hamstrings, butt, and lower back. I've chosen the Romanian deadlift for you because of your body type. It will allow you to take advantage of your long levers. It will make you a stronger runner in addition to tightening up the back of your legs and butt.

Jenny: Sounds interesting, but a little scary. I don't want my legs to bulk up lifting heavy weights.

Jon: I understand you don't want to get big, bulky muscles. The reality, though, is that most women don't have the levels of testosterone that men do that would create those big muscles. Judging from your build, I don't think it would be possible for you to bulk up even if you wanted to! [I make a note to send her an article about the same subject the next day.]

Jenny: Okay, I feel better. So, what's the clean and press?

Jon: The clean and press is a dynamic power exercise. It trains your entire body to be more explosive and has a great metabolic benefit. There isn't a muscle on your body that doesn't get worked! The clean and press will teach your body to transfer force well and burn a ton of calories. These two exercises, the dead lift and clean and press, are what I'm going to base your progression on. If you get good at them, I guarantee that you will become a better runner and put on lots of lean muscle.

Jenny: That sounds great. I'm excited to try them. What about the rest of the workout though? There is no way we're only doing those two exercises.

Jon: True. I want to put special emphasis on those two exercises since they're most important to you right now. The rest of your workout will actually work to support and make you better at the deadlift and clean and press. Let's get out there and I'll take you through the first day of your new workouts so you can see what I mean.

Jenny: Sounds good.

Do you see how this conversation used the Excitation System? Doing so, I accomplished the following things:

- I congratulated her on the work that she'd already done.
- I reaffirmed her goals of getting stronger at running and build-ing lean muscle. This helped refocus Jenny after we'd spent the past few weeks addressing her imbalances.
- I "closed the door" on the myth of weight lifting creating bulky muscles in women.
- I painted a clear picture of what the next phase of her training would look like, and why I chose it.
- I got her excited about working hard on the primary exercises.

I kept the conversation brief because she was relatively new to train-ing. If I described the ins and outs of a power program she might have been overwhelmed. If she had more experience, I might have done that.

Note that I also didn't describe any secondary or tertiary exercises. Jenny was pain-free and moving well after the 6-week anatomical adap-tation phase of training, so there weren't any other aspects I needed to put particular emphasis on. Otherwise, I would have addressed it and described the secondary or tertiary exercise I included to fix it.

I knew that Jenny would love the power training and would learn the secondary and tertiary exercises in due time. All I wanted from this brief conversation was for her to refocus and buy in to the program. If I hadn't taken the 5 minutes with her early on, she may have always been tentative about lifting heavy weights. I've found it's easier to convince a client to do something in the office ahead of time than on the gym floor.

Sometimes your excitation conversation will be long and involved and sometimes it will be brief. Regardless, take some time to get your client's buy-in before starting the workout.

TRAINING TIP:

The 5 or 10 minutes you take to properly educate your clients on their up-coming workouts will save you (and them!) time and frustration later on.

Keeping the Big Picture in Mind

If you want to use the Excitation System successfully, you should continually refer back to the big picture, or the client's overall goals. When you describe an exercise, explain why that will help your client reach her goals, which helps make each exercise experience emotional for her.

Often a new client cannot perform a difficult exercise right away, but that doesn't mean you can't get her excited about it. Let's say I have a client who can't yet do a deadlift. I'll say something like, "Since your goal is to tone your lower body, I want you deadlifting. The deadlift is one of the most effective exercises for your hamstrings, butt, and lower back. You're at a large mechanical advantage in the movement meaning that you'll be able to move a lot of weight, and that will lead to great gains. But right now the deadlift is too dangerous for you. We need to improve your mobility and activate your glutes first, so we're going to work on glutes activation work, dynamic flexibility, and core stability first. In addition, I'm going to be giving you variations of other exercises with a focus on grip strength so that later on you'll smash the exercise!"

This short speech educates the client on progression, and exposes her to my long-term vision and creates excitement to get there. This brief speech is just one part of the equation. I never stop working on their excitement.

Every exercise that I include in my programs has a function, and I make sure that clients know that. So, if I were having my above client performing a farmer's walk, I would describe the exercise and explain how the increased grip strength and core stability will help when she's performing a deadlift later on.

Once the day finally comes when my client is ready to perform a deadlift, I make a big deal about it! After all, she's worked hard to get to that point. I tell her the day before to help her mentally prepare for it, and get her excited. And after she's completed the first set, I reiterate all of the work that we've done leading up to it. I remind her about the specific parts of her journey that have led up to now. This helps make the experience emotional for her, and hopefully creates an "aha!" moment.

TRAINING TIP:

Always let your clients know how proud you are when they accomplish major steps toward their goals.

Inside Info – Mike Mahler

Mike Mahler is an authority on kettlebell training and the author of *Live Life Aggresively! What Self Help Gurus Should Be Telling You.*

Mike worked in sales and business development before getting laid off in 2002. Around that time he attended a kettlebell certification course taught by Pavel Tsatsouline (a kettlebell expert). After the course he decided that kettlebell training was going to be his focus in developing his fitness business.

Mike is a unique case in that he never worked for a gym. Early on in his career he did private training before transitioning to workshops, writing articles, and online consulting. He still teaches kettlebell workshops internationally and lectures on hormone optimization.

Mike markets through his website, social media, an online magazine, and a variety of publications and fitness radio shows.

Mike's 3 keys to succeeding as a personal trainer are:

1. You actually have to love working out yourself – If you don't, then get out of the business.

2. You have to have a genuine interest in helping others – Don't do it for recognition or big bucks. Those things will follow if you love training and helping others.

3. Learn the business side of things – Take marketing courses and read marketing books.

Mike's words to live by:

"Pick a focus rather than just being a generalist. Decide what you want to teach and exactly what kind of clients are a fit for you."

Mike Mahler is the owner of Mahler's Aggressive Strength. He's authored two books and taught over 100 kettlebell workshops. His website is www.mikemahler.com

Your Clients' Goals are Key

One of the reasons the Excitation System is so effective is because it continually reminds your clients that their workouts are helping them achieve their goals. To create workout plans to do that, you must know what your clients' goals are! That's why the first thing I do when sitting down with new clients is ask about their goals. Then I close my mouth and listen.

What I've found is that 99 percent of the time, my clients' stated goals are vague. Women usually want to lose fat or get toned. Men want to gain muscle or "get that v-shaped look." Well, new clients have no idea as to the timeline of a proper exercise program so they need to be educated on the process.

While plenty of gyms, articles, blogs, and books extol the virtue of "SMART" (Specific, Measurable, Attainable, Realistic, Time-oriented) goals, I've found that for a large percentage of clients, setting specific short- and long-term goals doesn't work. In addition, taking the time to work on goals uses up valuable face-to-face time with a client. Lastly, goal-setting often sets the trainer up for disaster if clients don't achieve their goals. You may be blamed for something that isn't within your control.

That's why I suggest you start with a full assessment to know what you're dealing with. Then educate your client about what your plan is for him or her, using the Excitation System.

Depending on the client, I will either devise a 3-month plan that includes specific goals or a 3-month plan that instead focuses on feeling or function.

I'll set specific goals with clients for several reasons. First, the client has made the conscious decision to start a program (which is often daunting) and therefore has the intrinsic motivation necessary to keep with it through thick and thin. Also, a client will make her greatest improvements early on. If your client's goal is fat loss, with a new exercise program and some small dietary changes, she should easily drop 5 to 10 pounds within the first month. If a client's goal is strength gain, the neurological component will be responsible for huge gains in the first 6 to 10 weeks on a resistance training program.

It's imperative that you educate clients on the physiology of these initial changes. If you don't, they may hold you accountable when they don't continually see the incredible improvements they made early on. I make sure to tell clients that while the initial improvements were large in an absolute sense, smaller improvements later become more significant in a relative sense. After 3 months, we usually avoid spending time setting specific goals and focus instead on the workouts themselves.

With other clients, however, I avoid specific goals and focus instead on feeling or function. I'll use this kind of program when a client scores poorly on an assessment or is coming to me post-rehabilitation. I explain that at this point in her training, the most important thing is to deal with her injury or imbalance. Later, the conditioning will take place. If you do choose to give goals based on function, I advise you to use a well-respected assessment tool that is used by professionals in different specialities.

As a trainer, I would rather spend that valuable time using my expertise to teach the client proper form and technique rather than inventing a number or goal for them to shoot for. That having been said, if your client is an athlete preparing for competition or has strong self-efficacy, goal-setting may be a valuable tool.

But usually this isn't the case and that's why the client has decided to hire you. Clients who have progressed beyond the initial 3 months should have enough self-efficacy to get them by without specific goal-setting. They've successfully started a program and completed the daunting task of sticking with it, and should have also achieved some measurable results.

That's why I think goal-setting isn't as important as some trainers think it is. I'm not saying that the client doesn't need to see continual progression, but proper monitoring of any good program should enable you to show that.

TRAINING TIP:

After the initial 3-month period, motivation becomes less of an issue for clients and goal-setting with the primary goal of encouragement goes down in importance.

So What's the Answer?

I hope that I've made a valid argument against goal-setting beyond the 3-month mark. But you may be asking, then what's the solution? How do you keep you clients engaged and committed, not just to exercise, but also to you?

My answer is to combine the power of workout monitoring and emotion. It's important to educate clients on the physiology of adaptation. Clients will get huge gains early with seemingly little work, but as they become more advanced, their gains become more significant but fewer in number.

Every step should be documented. Show clients their workout charts and note improvements. Take 5 minutes every 4 weeks to show them their results. First, they'll be blown away by all the work that they've done. It's a great feeling looking back at all of the numbers and reminiscing about the previous workouts.

"Aha!" moments also work well. Depending on the client, you can joke about how ridiculously easy earlier workouts feel now. Give them a point of reference for how far they've come.

As time goes by, your clients will have specific events that they want to work out for like a wedding, class reunion, or vacation. It's great to have an end goal for clients, and a good way to keep them engaged is to set a plan to *specifically* train towards this event. You can have some fun with it by using buzzwords or phrases such as working out to "get ripped for the beach." In addition to helping them maintain focus, they'll have another thing to talk to their friends about—the awesome beach body workout you're putting them through!

TRAINING TIP:

Keep clients motivated by continually monitoring their progress, and using specific events as training motivators.

POINTS TO REMEMBER:

- Your real job as a trainer is to get your clients excited about training.
- Your clients' goals should always determine the workouts you choose—and they should understand that.
- Specific goal-setting can be an effective tool in the short term, but is less important than motivating clients with "aha!" moments.

Chapter 7

Keep it Simple: The Focus System and Why it Works

"Try again. Fail again. Fail better."

- SAMUEL BECKETT

Search for the word "workouts" on Google, and you'll get more than 11,000,000 hits. Search for "training program" and you'll get more than 370,000,000 hits. So how do you decide *which* workout or training program to follow?

You probably became a personal trainer because you love fitness, but that doesn't mean you know how to train someone. You've trained yourself, but now you're responsible for training a huge variety of clients. In fact, my clients range from 25-67 years old. Some are athletic; others are obese. Some clients are injury-free while others have pain with any movement.

So how do I devise workouts for beginners, regardless of background? The answer? Keep it simple. In this chapter you'll learn how to follow the Focus System to create a training program for clients new to exercise. The type of workout program you use may vary, but use the Focus System (and the Excitation System, which is described in chapter 6) and you'll have the foundation to train clients safely and effectively. It's beyond the scope of this book to teach you proper programming and exercise selection. What I will do is show you my system for quickly and effectively designing workouts from start to finish.

Understanding the Physiology of Skill Acquisition

Before we talk about proper exercise instruction, let's review the basics of skill acquisition. Nobody will pick up any movement or skill right away, especially not one as difficult as the squat or clean and press. You must also remember that a lot of your clients will have muscle imbalances due to the repetitive nature of many of the things we do throughout the day. Muscles responsible for repetitive movements may be strong while opposing muscles are weak and/or tight. Therefore you need to "reprogram" your clients and, in the words of Dr. Stu McGill, "groove movement patterns," or stretch the overused muscles and strengthen the underused muscles while teaching the proper movements.

When grooving a client's movement patterns, keep the reps low and make sure that he maintains proper form. The moment his form breaks, he should stop the exercise. If your client is having trouble picking up one particular part of the exercise, then don't allow him to continue. Stop him, have him visualize the proper form, and then re-adjust.

For example, consider a client who is having a hard time retracting his scapula during the seated row, which is common for anybody with postural issues. I demonstrate the exercise with good form pointing out major cues. If I see my client is having trouble, I will physically guide their shoulders into the proper position.

I then ask the client to stop and think about how it felt when his shoulders were moving properly as I guided him through the movement. After he's visualized the motion and knows what it feels like to do the movement properly, I have him try again. The second his form breaks, I tell him to stop, visualize, readjust, and try again. It is through this concentrated repetition that skills are learnt quickly and effectively.

Let me get technical for a moment. We improve specific skills by increasing the myelination of the nerve fiber, which occurs when supporter cells called oligodendrocytes and astrocytes wrap more myelin on the nerve fiber, which improves nerve transmission. This means that the nerve becomes better insulated, and increased insulation in the nerve means that electrical impulses are faster and more effective. From a fitness standpoint, that added insulation makes your movements smoother and more automatic.

The best way to add myelination and therefore improve the effectiveness of the nerve transmission is to *fail with purpose*. In other words, keep trying and visualizing the move properly and it will become automatic.

Failing better is the goal, but clients usually don't understand that. So I suggest you educate your clients about the physiology of skill acquisition and remind them that this process takes time. I spend a lot of time with new clients making sure that they understand why I'm not letting them work as hard as they want. It's sometimes difficult because when new clients are sold on personal training, they're excited and raring to go. But take the time to teach proper form. Once they learn how to do a move well, proper form will be cemented into their brains.

TRAINING TIP:

Failing with purpose leads to effective skill development. Encourage proper form early on and make sure that your clients understand its importance.

Inside Info – Brad Schoenfeld

Brad Schoenfeld has over 400,000 books in print, 8+ different titles. He is widely regarded as one a leading authority on body composition training.

Brad originally obtained a bachelors degree and followed it up with a medical imaging certificate from vocational school. He worked at a family medical business, earned a master's degree in exercise science, and is working towards his doctorate.

His fitness career started with a short stint doing in-home training. He found it inefficient and opened his own facility. Most of his time is now spent teaching at the college/graduate level and conducting workshops for fitness professionals.

The majority of his marketing has been through word of mouth, appearances in major media and through his blog.

Brad's 3 keys to succeeding as a personal trainer are:

1. Be knowledgeable – Everything starts with good knowledge of the science of exercise. If you don't know what you're doing, you not only won't get people proper results, you could hurt them. You need to be a student of the craft, constantly seeking to acquire more knowledge. Read the research. Go to conferences. Further your education. Learning never stops, no matter how much schooling you've had.

2. Communicate effectively – No matter how knowledgeable you are, you won't be a good trainer unless you communicate properly with your clients. The essence of communication is listening. Learn to be a good listener, and you're halfway there. The other half is knowing what motivates your client and responding in a manner that will inspire.

3. Have confidence – When you train a client, confidence is paramount. If a client senses you aren't confident in your approach, you're done. It's imperative that everything you do is done with conviction. Sadly, a lot of bad trainers are very successful because they ooze confidence.

Brad's words to live by:

"If you are good and you display confidence, you have a leg up on most"

Brad Schoenfeld M.Sc., C.S.C.S. is a popular fitness author and educator. He maintains a blog at www.workout911.com.

Introduction to the Focus System

I developed the Focus System after years of research on the physiology of skill acquisition and tested it for years. I've found that it helps clients pick up movements quickly, and understand why they're performing different exercises. Once you know your client's goals [see chapter 4], you can devise a program for him.

The Focus System is based on the fact that most of your clients will be beginners. (As the client becomes more advanced, there are hundreds of different training protocols to choose from depending on his goals, and more advanced programming might be needed.) But you'll find that for most clients, especially those new to exercise, the Focus System is the perfect training tool. It's composed of 6-steps:

1. Decide what rep range is most appropriate for the client's goals.
2. Pick 2 to 4 exercises that are the **most important** for that client to reach his primary goal, keeping his initial assessment in mind. Rep range will dictate the type of exercise.
3. Pick accessory (secondary) movements that will help the client develop skill and strength on the primary exercises.
4. Pick rehab (tertiary) exercises depending on the client's existing injuries, limitations, or imbalances. If no injury or imbalance exists, pick "prehab" exercises to strengthen commonly injured areas with their specific type of training or body type.
5. Decide on an appropriate cardio protocol.
6. Put together an effective dynamic warm-up, including myofascial release, keeping in mind the client's skill level and comfort in the gym.

Now let's take a closer look at each of these steps:

Rep Range (The Great Decider)
Right away after establishing your client's goals, you should know what rep range he should be working in. If your client is training for

power, his rep range will be 1 to 5; if he's training for muscular endurance, 12 to 15; and so on.

The rep range dictates every aspect of the workout:

- The number of sets is determined by rep range. For example, if the client is training for power in the 1-5 range, he will be completing more sets of the primary exercises. On the other hand, an endurance protocol of 12-15 reps will require fewer sets for a training effect. Efficiency of movement is also less important when the goal is muscular endurance. There is less of a focus on perfect form and neurological fatigue isn't as much of an issue as it is with a power workout.

- Rep range will also dictate the type of exercise that you will include. For a workout with 1-5 reps, you'll opt for power exercises such as the clean and press over something like the biceps curl. I do appreciate the need to perform power training on isolated muscle groups for certain sports, but that's not the norm for the average client's power workout.

- Tempo, to a degree, is also determined by rep range. A power exercise may include a 10X (1 second eccentric, 0 second pause, performed as quickly as possible) tempo. To improve muscular endurance, a number of different tempos can be useful. Pausing under tension will increase the stress on the muscle and is a good way to push the client that extra 10 percent. The most common tempo that's used for muscle gain is the "3011," or 3 seconds during the eccentric phase of the lift, 0 seconds pause, 1 second for the concentric phase, and 1 second pause.

- Rest intervals are also determined by rep range. A power reps range of 1-5 will require 2-3 minutes to replenish the creatine phosphate system. Your goal is to train the client at efficiency, so training when a client's creatine system is depleted is counterproductive. Muscular endurance, on the other hand, requires much shorter rest intervals. The goal is to improve the client's recovery so you need to stress both the anaerobic and aerobic systems.

TRAINING TIP:

After establishing your client's goals, determine what rep range is appropriate. Then you can use any textbook or training program to determine which exercises to include in his program.

Primary Exercises

To choose the primary exercises, I use a combination of intuition and knowledge. An analysis of the client's body type, in combination with their goals and assessment will dictate the *most important* exercises. These exercises are exclusively large multi-joint exercises and are often some variation of the squat, deadlift, lunge, chin up, row, chest press, or power movement (clean and press etc.).

The primary exercises are the focus of the workout, and they're what the client will get the most gains from. Therefore I base progression of the client's workouts on the primary exercises. If they're getting stronger at the front squat, I don't need to know how their leg extension is doing. (Of course I still track the weights and reps of all the exercises in the workout.)

There are two reasons I put so much emphasis on the primary exercises. First, beginner clients cannot get good at more than 2-4 exercises at once. Giving them too many exercises means that clients won't learn proper form and won't be able to progress efficiently. Second, it's much easier to sell a client on 2 exercises rather than 20. You don't want to overwhelm your client, especially if he's new to working out.

For a power workout, using the 2 above rep range examples, 2 primary exercises might be the sumo deadlift and bench press. For a muscular endurance workout, 2 primary exercises might be the goblet squat and seated row.

Secondary Exercises

The secondary movements are where I have the greatest flexibility and the most fun. Often I'll program these exercises as supersets or circuits. I'm not as picky about form as I am with the primary exercises. At this point in the workout, the client will be neurologically and physically tired since the primary exercises take constant focus.

You have the biggest variance with the exercise selection here. The purpose of the secondary exercises is to support the primary and take the client one step closer to his goal. This is where I'll include things like single joint movements, abdominal work (rotation, flexion, anti-rotation), and single-leg exercises.

In a power workout where the primary exercises are the sumo deadlift and bench press, I might choose barbell glutes bridges and dumbbell skull crushers as secondary exercises. For the muscular endurance workout where the primary exercises are the goblet squat and seated row, the secondary exercises might be a single-leg squat and dumbbell cross-body hammer curl.

Tertiary Exercises

You can use tertiary exercises in two different places during the workout. They can be used either as active rest between sets or after the secondary exercises if there is time left in the workout. Often I'll have some prehab exercises on hand if time allows.

When I originally designed the Focus System, I considered tertiary exercises to be purely rehabilitative in nature, but I've now expanded the term to include "prehab" exercises. Prehab exercises are to prevent injuries, not treat them. They vary depending on the different stresses that primary exercises place on the body. That having been said, some clients will need enough rehabilitation that you won't be able to fit in prehab work.

Tertiary exercises aren't impacted by the type of workout your client is doing. If the client needs to fix an imbalance, for example, it doesn't matter whether he's training for power or muscular endurance.

Cardio

I'm not a big proponent of steady-state cardio. It's an important aspect of fitness, but I've found that you can often program sufficient cardio into a resistance training routine. Remember that the cardio protocol you prescribe has to fall in line with your client's goals. Cardio can be counterproductive if improperly programmed; for example, a hypertrophy workout shouldn't have much, if any, steady state cardio. You can be good at putting on muscle and cardio at the same time but you can't be great at both.

For a power program, a cardio protocol might be 1-2 days/week of HIIT (high intensity interval training). For muscular endurance training, I would suggest a combination of steady state running with hill or interval training.

Dynamic Warm-up and Myofascial Release

The dynamic warm-up depends on the client's skill and comfort level. A beginner client will probably be reluctant to do a long dynamic warm-up alone. If the client is more confident, I'll give him a warm-up complete with dynamic stretching and self myofascial release, or foam rolling, to help increase blood flow. I go through it once with him and then give him a handout, asking him to complete the full warm-up before we begin training.

The warm-up will depend on the nature of the workout. For example, a power workout will likely have more hip and shoulder mobility drills, and more myofascial release. A muscular endurance workout's warm-up will include fewer individual dynamic stretches and focus on increasing blood flow throughout the body. In addition, I might opt to do the myofascial release at the end of the workout to massage out any knots and help break down scar tissue in overused muscles.

Using the Focus System

Now that you know the 6 steps of the Focus System, let's take a look at how you would use it with a client. I introduce every primary exercise with the following 5-step process:

1. Show the client the name of the exercise on paper and repeat it aloud.
2. Explain why I chose the exercise specifically for the client.
3. Make it relevant to the client in terms of his goals or experience (the more personal you can make this, the better).
4. Demonstrate the exercise, highlighting the 2 most important points for proper form. (If clients often make a common mistake, point that out as well.)
5. Have the client try the exercise.

I only follow these steps for the primary exercises as it's a time-consuming process and you don't want to risk your client losing focus. For all other exercises, I follow steps 4 and 5—unless I have a specific tertiary exercise for rehab or prehab. In that case, additional detail is necessary.

So, here's what that a conversation introducing a primary exercise might sound like with my client, Bill. Bill had experienced chronic low back pain in the past but he was pain-free and I knew he was ready to step up to the next level of training. I'd told him that in advance so he knew what to expect. I also asked him to perform a full dynamic warm-up before we met, and to meet me in my office.

Jon: Hi, Bill. How are things going today?

Bill: Great. I feel good today, but I'm a little nervous about the next stage.

Jon: Don't be nervous at all. You wouldn't be progressing if you weren't ready. As you know, we've been doing a lot of dynamic flexibility work and fixing up your movement patterns. We'll continue that but that training will be secondary from here on out. I've been really happy that your back is feeling good again and you've started to trim down, but we're now going to accelerate the fat burning.

Bill: Great.

Jon: I've chosen two main exercises for you that are going to get you great results. They are the Clean and Press and Squat. I've chosen these two exercises specifically for you because they both have the ability to burn a lot of fat. They work a lot of large muscles, so you'll get a great metabolic effect from them. In addition, they both force you to keep a stable core so you'll get good ab training and they'll strengthen your back as well.

Bill: Interesting. What about the rest of the workout?

Jon: The rest of the workout is secondary. I want to put particular emphasis on these 2 exercises because I'm basing your progression on them. I chose these two exercises specifically because if you improve on these 2 exercises, then I promise you'll get stronger and lose fat. The other exercises throughout this workout will either be a continuation of our low back/posture regime or help support clean and press and squat.

Bill: So which are we starting with? I'm ready!

Jon: [I demonstrate the squat to Bill.] As you sit back in the squat, it's important to press into your heels. This will shift the weight back to your glutes and hamstrings. As you're pressing back up I want you to breathe out and squeeze your butt at the top. Why don't you try it out?

At this point I have Bill try the movement with the barbell alone. I then correct the technique as needed until he has the proper form down. (Note that the cues I used for the squat are examples. I know different trainers have different ways of teaching moves. Regardless of how you teach, though, choose only 1 or 2 cues while you demonstrate good form. A picture paints a thousand words so a good demonstration is more important than tons of cues. After he's done a couple reps, you can make any corrections and have your client try again.)

This brief conversation with Bill accomplished several things. I complimented Bill on the good work that he's already done, citing specific examples. Next, I reinforced his goals and highlighted what he's already done to achieve them. I gave him a week's warning to get him chomping at the bit. By the time I introduced the squat, my explanation was brief and to the point. Usually clients just want an overview of what they're doing and why they're doing it. Therefore I recommend you keep your explanations brief unless prompted further.

TRAINING TIP:

Don't get wrapped up in describing exercises—all you need to include are the major points. After the client tries the exercise, you can identify what he needs to change and cue him accordingly.

Training Traps to Avoid

I'd like to close this chapter by mentioning some common "training traps" to avoid. As a trainer, your focus should always be on helping your clients get results. Avoid training traps like the following:

- **Program-hopping**. Too often trainers deviate from their plan because they've gotten excited about a new method of training. The best results can often be found with a relentless devotion to the basics. For example, I knew a trainer, Paul, who was working with a client, Jeff, who wanted to lose fat and put on muscle. They agreed that Jeff would add muscle mass first, and then focus on burning fat, and Paul created a program with those goals in mind. A month into training, Jeff was looking and feeling good, but then Paul decided to have Jeff do Tabata training (a high-intensity interval workout) instead. At the 3-month assessment, Jeff hadn't come near to his original agreed-upon goals. Paul had fallen into the trap of program hopping and Jeff's results suffered. If Paul had stuck with hypertrophy training for the full 3 months, Jeff would have met his goals. (In addition,

Jeff would have gained a lot more from the Tabata training during the next phase of his training with the added muscle mass.)

- **Progressing too quickly.** More often than not, your client is new to exercise or has been exercising improperly. That's why he came to you. Your job is to devise a plan that works for that client. A simple program that works is better than a fancy, complicated one that doesn't! Linear progression works best for beginner clients and complicated loading schemes should be saved for when a client becomes more advanced.

- **Lack of a long-term vision.** It's hard to get your client focused without a long-term vision for him. This vision gets the client excited about what he's specifically going to accomplish, and gives you direction. *Everything* you do as a trainer should be directed towards this long-term goal, which will form the basis of your progression planning. For example, if a client wants to burn fat you can progress them towards metabolic training and work towards barbell complexes, which build muscle and increase metabolism. Just remember the goal every step of the way and continue to lead the client towards it.

- **Using too many toys.** Don't get obsessed with fitness toys. More companies are trying to capitalize on the booming fitness market by putting out new equipment, but in my experience, the tried and tested basics always work best. I can't think of a better tool for burning fat than a barbell. Having a wide range of exercises and equipment at your disposal is a great idea. Just think of it as your training toolbox. You must understand the benefits and downfalls of the gadgets at your disposal, and when to use them. (For more suggestions on training tools and techniques, visit www.theptdc.com.)

- **Information overload.** This can lead to program hopping, which I already discussed above. There are tools ranging from dumbbells to cables to steps to BOSU balls to cables, and you can find hundreds of new exercises on the Internet in just minutes. Don't be overwhelmed by information overload; as I said before, often the tried and tested work best. Of course sometimes you'll discover a new exercise that serves a purpose for your client. It's your job to be the detective and determine whether a new exercise is worth incorporating into a program.

The main point I want you to remember is that you should always keep your client's goals in mind. What do you hope the program will accomplish? Does every single one of the exercises you included bring your client closer to *their* goals in some way? If you can't explain to the client why you chose a particular exercise, leave it out no matter how nice it looks.

TRAINING TIP:

You should always be able to explain why you chose every exercise in a client's program.

When Clients Ask About the "Latest Thing"

There will always be an endless supply of new fitness products, videos, and books that promise to be the "next big thing." Tune into television at night and you'll see infomercials that support their claims with studies and experts. They are usually marketed as giving results more quickly, with less effort, and for a bargain price.

People will ask your opinion about the newest hit product or workout video, so stay up-to-date on what's popular and what's being marketed to consumers. If I've already researched something, I'll share that with the person. If I don't know about the program, I'll look into it and then get back to the person asking for the information.

When I'm asked about a product or program, I don't bash it. I try to point out the positives and the negatives. Say a client asks me about a new workout that his friend has had success with, I might say, "I'm familiar with that workout, and I know people who have done it. It's a good plan but there's nothing magical about it. If anyone exercises at a high intensity, following a proper program including appropriate progression and rest, and eats a clean diet for 3 months, he'll get results. Any good trainer will be the first to tell you that consistency with appropriate progression is imperative in getting results, and he's packaged his product so that people will buy it. I wish that I had thought of it first!

"That having been said, I also know a lot of people that haven't been successful on this program for a variety of reasons. One is that people aren't accountable to anyone but themselves, so it requires a lot of intrinsic motivation. Second, the workout isn't designed for each individual, which means anyone with an injury should be extremely careful. And you probably already know that no workout can match what you get working one-on-one with a trainer."

See what I mean? I haven't put down the product, but I've pointed out the positives and negatives from an educated point of view. I've found that clients are usually always nervous about trying out new products but they do want to be informed. If you're worried that a client will leave you for an infomercial product, I suggest you provide more personalized service and start going the extra 10 percent!

If you haven't heard of the product or workout before, take quick action. Make a note and do your research so you can provide your client with solid articles about the product or your opinion about it as soon as possible. The longer a product or workout has been around, the higher the chance you'll find articles, blog posts, and other information about it online. Read with a critical eye and form your own educated opinion.

TRAINING TIP:

Stay up-to-date on the latest workouts and fitness programs, and be prepared to tell clients the advantages and downfalls about them.

POINTS TO REMEMBER:

- Using the Focus System with clients helps keep their motivation high and keeps them from becoming overwhelmed by a workout routine.

- Every exercise you give a client should have a specific purpose— and the client should understand that.

- New fitness toys, products, and programs come along all the time, but usually the "tried and tested" approach is the best to take.

Chapter 8

Fuel for the Fire: Keeping Clients Inspired

"The most powerful weapon on earth is the human soul on fire."

- FERDINAND FOCH

In the preceding 3 chapters, you learned how to create a relationship with new clients and how to use the Excitation System and Focus System with them. That knowledge alone will let you launch a promising career. But for long-term success as a trainer, you must be able to maintain long-term clients—and that means being able to motivate and inspire them for weeks, months, or even years.

What works for one client won't work for another, but there are some effective ways to keep clients excited about and motivated to keep working out—and hopefully, continuing to train with you. I've found that some strategies tend to work better with extroverted or outgoing clients while others are more effective with introverted ones.

Know your Clients

In chapter 9, you'll learn about some of the common personality types you're likely to encounter when training and how to work with them. The most important thing you can do to help motivate any particular client, however, is to understand him or her. Is your client shy or outgoing? What does she do for a living? What is her family situation? (Is she married or single, for example? Does she have children at home?) What kinds of activities does she enjoy in her spare time? The more information you have about your client and what makes her tick, the better able you are to connect with her. Here are some techniques that can maintain motivation and increase client retention:

- **Exercise contracts**. Exercise contracts detail their commitment both to you and their program and have a start and end date. These can be especially effective with introverted clients as the contracts make them accountable without having to involve anyone else. If you use contracts, both you and your client should sign it to show that you too are committed to their goals. Keep one copy for yourself and give one to your client. The contract also is a "take-away" that clients may show to other people.
- **Rewards**. Rewards can be big motivators. You might offer either free sessions or a refund of some of their money once they reach their goal. Or you can make the reward a gift card to the client's favourite store, a T-shirt, or gym bag. I opt for fitness-related gifts with my logo on them. I also give out a monthly award to the client who has reached a major goal, overcome some adversity, or simply worked extremely hard that month. The client gets a custom-made badge and I write them up on my website as well.
- **Journaling**. Plenty of studies show that keeping a journal helps people stick to their workout routines. Encourage clients to keep a book or calendar detailing their workouts and progress, or give them a workout log with your logo on it. You can also

print up a copy of the client's completed workouts and give it to the client as a gift so he can see how far he's come.

- **Fitness tests**. If you have "type A" clients who like to achieve specific goals, fitness tests can be a great motivator. They work harder so they won't fail the upcoming tests; just be sure to help them set reasonable goals.
- **Workout partners**. Organizing a signup board at your gym for workout partners can keep clients motivated and enhance the community at your gym. If you have two clients doing similar workouts on their own, introduce them and suggest they work out together. They're more likely to stick with their routine.
- **Star system**. My grade 2 teacher gave us a gold star every time we did something well or answered a question in class. I'm proud to say that I was the proud owner of a genuine leather cowboy wallet at the end of the year for winning that game. Though the wallet was great, it was not my motivation. My motivation stemmed from looking up at that board every day and seeing my classmates get stars along with me. I knew I had to get my homework done and answer some questions the following day to stay ahead. My point? Consider using a "star system" or other visible tool at your gym. Post your clients' names on a board, give them gold stars when they do something great, and give the winner a prize.
- **Self-analysis**. To stay tuned in to my clients' need, I use an evaluation form after they've trained with me for a while. The form asks questions like:
  1. Why did you originally join our club?
  2. What were some of your original motivations and why did you choose me?
  3. Did you ever feel like quitting? Why? What made you stay?
  4. Did you have "aha" moments? What were they?
  5. How can I (or the club) make your experience even better and help you progress towards even more impressive goals?

Answering these questions helps clients learn about their own motivators, which can develop self-efficacy, which is discussed more below.

- **Social support**. Giving clients printouts of their workouts, articles about their goals or injuries, and a detailed plan can help build motivation. The takeaways also give your clients something to talk about with their loved ones, which can help them get support and may result in referrals as well.

- **Surprise them**. One of the simplest but most effective ways to motivate clients is to send cards. I send cards for the holidays, on birthdays, and when clients reach their goals, but you don't even need a special occasion. I buy nice cards as I want my clients to display them at home or work, which can lead to more referrals!

- **Compliments**. Compliments can be incredibly powerful. When used effectively, they can reinforce positive habits. For a compliment to be effective, it must be sincere, specific, and timed properly. A compliment about a client's personal appearance, like commenting about new workout clothing or a new haircut, is appropriate because it shows that you pay close attention to him or her. (I've noticed that clients will often start wearing more form-fitting workout clothes as they get in better shape.) Be careful not to compliment clients too often, which can appear fake. I give quick "well dones" and fist bumps when training a client, but I save my big compliments for special occasions, like when a client has really struggled with a particular movement. For example, I had a client who had been training for weeks before he was able to complete 5 reps of barbell squats with excellent form. When he did so, I said, "Great job! You kept a nice strong back on the way down, and didn't have any forward shift coming up. You were definitely focusing on driving through your heels. I can't tell you how happy this makes me to see you squat so well. Remember when you started out and your knees hurt even as you sat down? I'm proud of you." Note that this compliment was specific, personal, and focused on what he had achieved. A sincere compliment that points out how far your client has come also helps him develop intrinsic motivation.

TRAINING TIP:

Use sincere, specific compliments with clients for the greatest impact.

Helping Clients Develop Self-Efficacy

You've been learning about ways to help motivate your clients, but the real key to motivation comes from internal, not external sources. When your clients develop self-efficacy, they will be motivated from the inside out. As a trainer, you should understand the concept of self-efficacy and know how to help your clients develop it—it will enhance their experience in the gym so they see results more quickly.

Self-efficacy is defined as the belief that you have the ability to execute the course of action required to manage prospective situations. In other words, you know you can do it, whatever "it" is. Canadian psychologist Albert Bandura, Ph.D. developed the concept of self-efficacy and has studied and written about it for years. He describes 4 major sources of it:

- **Social modelling.** This is achieved by witnessing others accomplish a similar task. If your client sees or knows others who have accomplished their goals, rehabbed their injuries, or become comfortable in the gym, for example, your client will become more confident *he* can succeed. Social modelling is especially effective if the client knows the "model" personally.

- **Social persuasion**. This comes in the form of verbal encouragement, such as with effective complimenting. The client will have less self-doubt and start to believe in himself more and more.
- **Psychological responses**. This aspect of self-efficacy has to do with a client's reaction to certain situations, such as trying a new exercise. Helping your client elevate his mood and lower his stress before a workout can help lessen negative psychological responses that may interfere with developing self-efficacy. (Note that the intensity of the psychological responses is *secondary* to how it's perceived and interpreted. In other words, you can help a client understand that an elevated heart rate can be a sign that his body is getting ready to take on a new challenge.)
- **Mastery experiences**. This is perhaps the most important aspect of Bandura's model as far as personal training goes. When a client performs well, his self-efficacy increases. When he fails at something, it decreases. It's therefore important to allow your client to succeed often, and to make note of their successes, early on in training. The easiest way to provide a client with a mastery experience is to start them at the proper stage of progression within an exercise; in other words, give them a move and a weight that they can handle. If a client fails, don't dwell on it. Quickly shift focus and bring up a previous situation where that client succeeded. The goal is to get the client thinking about their failure for as little time as possible.

As a trainer, Bandura's self-efficacy research should always be in the back of your mind. Note that new clients will benefit more from its application than more seasoned clients since the more experienced ones have already gotten results. Their initial intrinsic motivation was strong enough for them to persevere through their original insecurities. As clients becomes more seasoned, they gain mastery experiences and likely experience social persuasion from friends and family.

Let me share several examples of how I've helped clients develop self-efficacy so you can see it in action. Remember my client Pam from chapter 5? Pam was apprehensive about working out, but the fact that her friend Cindy had already achieved great results helped Pam develop her own self-efficacy. That's an example of social modeling.

I'd been training with another client, Fred, for a year. He'd started out at 450 pounds. During that year, he'd lost 120 pounds, eliminated his knee pain, and regained his shoulder mobility, which was a huge problem for him early on. I decided to write an assisted pull-up into his program. I knew he was still heavy, but he had gained a lot of strength and I thought he would be able to do this exercise.

However, after instructing Fred on the Gravitron machine, Fred got stuck on the bottom and couldn't pull himself up. I quickly showed him how to safely step off the machine and set the weight to the easiest setting, but once again, Fred couldn't pull himself up. Fred was still too heavy for the assisted pull-up and I had to act fast. Without mentioning anything about the pull-up, I set a manageable weight on the lat pull-down machine and had him bang out a set.

I made a mistake with Fred by having him attempt an exercise that was too advanced for him. Avoid this whenever you can, especially for clients with low self-efficacy. Challenging more experienced trainees with advanced moves is another thing; because of their high confidence, a failure is less likely to affect their self-efficacy.

As a trainer, you're also likely to encounter clients who show up for a workout and immediately say that they feel fat, tired, or out of shape. By using social persuasion, you can relieve anxiety that would reduce a client's self-efficacy.

My client Jenny had had an original goal of losing 20 pounds, and had only lost 5 so far. However, she was finally comfortable with exercise and had achieved some results. So I was surprised when Jenny came in for a session and told me that she felt fat. She'd had some friends over to swim and felt self-conscious in her bathing suit.

I brought Jenny into my office so we could talk more. After listening to her, I reminded her about one of her previous aha moments. Two months earlier, she'd taken a cruise with her husband and had worn a flowing red dress, and her husband had told her how beautiful she looked. Then Jenny jumped in recalling how she had given away all of her jeans because they had all become too big for her. The emotional response that she gained from visualizing her red dress brought up other positive emotions!

After our brief conversation, I had Jenny do her warm-up. She had a great workout that day and left her "fat" feelings in the office.

Physical changes occur slowly, and clients' moods ebb and flow during that time. Some days they'll be happy and motivated to train. Other days, they may feel depressed, discouraged, or even angry. Pay attention to your clients' moods at the beginning of a session. To use social persuasion, let your client speak—even rant! Often your client just needs someone to listen to her frustrations. After she's gotten whatever she needs off her chest, encourage your client to remember and focus on aha moments. After she has done so, get her out on the gym floor and get her sweating!

TRAINING TIP:

You can use social modeling, social persuasion, mastery experiences, and psychological responses to help increase self-efficacy in clients. Make sure that new clients develop ample self-efficacy to help retain them.

Inside Info – Neghar Fonooni

Neghar Fonooni is the only female in Maryland, U.S.A. to hold both the RKC II and CK-FMS designations. She is a successful trainer and internet personality.

In 2000 Neghar started working at her local YMCA and quickly transitioned to working as a trainer when she realized she had a knack for coaching. At the time she was also studying journalism, so training was a hobby as opposed to a career choice.

Like many others, Neghar joined the military after 9/11. She graduated from college in 2003 and spent the next four years working as an Air Force Arabic Linguist. After serving, she returned to a full-time career training and writing.

Neghar has worked at the YMCA, Bally's Total Fitness, a large privately owned gym, a women's-only yoga studio, and a small 24-hour private facility. She now works in and manages a private performance training facility. Her days consist of coaching private, semi-private and group clientele.

Like many other top coaches, Neghar doesn't commit any finances to marketing. Instead, she writes a popular blog and maintains two websites. She has an extensive YouTube channel where she performs incredible feats of strength and instructs. She also uses Facebook as her marketing platform. She's been an independent contractor since 2007 and loves the freedom and flexibility that comes with it.

Neghar's 3 keys to succeeding as a personal trainer are:

1. Education - I am where I am today because I read a ton of books and attend seminars regularly. If you want to educate and inspire your clients, you must be educated and inspire yourself.
2. Passion and patience – These are two sides of the same coin. You must be passionate about movement and helping others, but you must also be patient and let them get there in their own time.
3. Time management – Burn out is common in this field. You must be in control of your schedule and manage your time properly or you'll quickly tire of the job. Learning to set boundaries is also important so as not to commit to things that may over extend you.

Neghar's words to live by:

"You can certainly make a decent living training clients 30-40 hours per week and stay there comfortably. For some people, that may be as far as they go. For others, there is an ambitious nature within them that will allow them to take their business much further. Being successful is dependent on how many people you reach."

Neghar Fonooni RKC II, CK-FMS is a Performance Training Specialist. She maintains a blog at www.negharfonooni.com.

Working with Uncommitted Clients

Few trainers consistently work with highly motivated individuals. If we did, our job might not exist! In modern day society, exercise's priority is placed far behind work, family, friends, social time, and sleep. It's usually fit in when convenient. As a trainer, you want to make it a higher priority for your clients.

You will encounter clients who seem to be uncommitted. They may miss appointments, show up late, or seem unengaged during your session. Your job is find out what the problem is, and help the client address it.

Ask whether the client has had a previous bad experience with a trainer. If so, make sure that you don't repeat the problem [see chapter 5 for more on this]. If the issue isn't a previous negative experience, it's likely a personal issue and is one of the following:

Unsupportive Spouse

I've dealt with this issue a number of times. The spouse may believe that a trainer is a frivolous expense or that their significant other's time would be better spent with the family or at work.

I suggest you provide your client with lots of written material on the importance of training in addition to a write-up of your short and long-term plan with the client. I also make myself available to meet with the client's spouse if he or she is willing. I also sit down with my client and get him to tell me why exercise is so important *for him*. Having him create an emotional attachment to exercise will encourage him to stand his ground when speaking with his spouse.

Lack of Community

A lack of positive relationships in the gym won't necessarily cause clients to leave, but good relationships will encourage them to stay. Your early days training a new client should include lots of introductions to other trainers and long-term members. Seeing familiar faces when they walk through the door goes a long way in increasing adherence.

Over the long term, this habit also creates a unique feel and works to position you better. When your clients feel at home in the gym, they're likely to train more often. They're also more likely to chat with new members and may recommend you to others.

Lack of Education

Clients may be uncommitted due to lack of education. If you're not able to explain *why* you're doing what you're doing [see chapter 7], they will eventually lose faith and leave.

It takes 6-8 weeks for any serious physical adaptation to take place in most new clients. Before that, clients are experiencing primarily neural gains. That's a lot of time and money for somebody who's been promised results and made the life changes necessary to start working with you. If you don't take the time to explain the process of adaption to your clients, you may lose them before they get real results.

To a new client, I might say something like, "You don't build a skyscraper without lots of planning and a strong foundation. It takes time, but the sky's the limit." Or I'll say, "The easiest way to imagine your fitness is as a large stone wheel. It will take a lot of momentum to get going, but once it starts moving, it's hard to slow down." The idea is to use a metaphor that your clients can relate to and remember.

If I feel a client would appreciate a more scientific approach, I'll get into the physiology of adaption in more detail. I'll say something like:

"I'd like to take a couple minutes to explain adaptation to you. The first couple months are called the anatomical adaptation phase. Here's what I mean by that: (I sketch the graph below and explain it as I go).

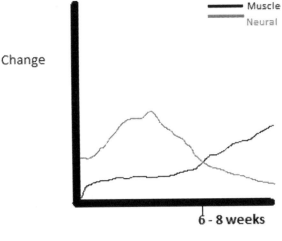

"As you can see, the first system that will start to adapt is the neuro-logical system. That happens rather quickly, so you will see strength gains within the first couple weeks. Somewhere around the 6–8 week mark, mus-cle gains start to happen and an overlap takes place. That's when you will start seeing the aesthetic benefits of your training.

"One other point to note is that connective tissue adapts slower than muscle. Therefore in the interest of safety, the weights may be a little lighter than you feel you can manage early on. I want to make sure your joints are protected. Not to worry though—the stimulus on your body will be more than adequate to have a strong training effect. Later on we will be getting more specific in your training to stimulate specific systems. For now, whole body training is the best course of action. Does that make sense?"

Remember that if you can't give your client a reason for doing a par-ticular exercise, you shouldn't do it. By keeping your clients' minds active throughout the workouts, they'll be more engaged in the training and will get better results. I also make sure to ask my more advanced clients their opinions on workouts and where they would like to head next. I then take the time to educate them on the pros and cons of their next goals in addition to what it will take to get them there to gain their buy-in to your training program.

Life Crises

Sometimes you don't know why a client is uncommitted, but going the extra 10 percent can make the difference. Take a trainer I worked with, who had been working with a client for 4 months when she started cancelling sessions out of the blue. He immediately sat his client down to speak about what was going on.

She told him that her husband had just been diagnosed with late-stage cancer and had been given 6 months to live. Her life was falling apart. The only time she was able to let loose a little was in the gym but she had no control over her schedule. This trainer came in as early as 5:30 a.m. and as late as 9:00 p.m. to train his client. He knew how important exercise was for her well-being and went the extra 10 percent to help her any way he could. He kept the client and, as a result of treating her so well, had other clients referred to him through her. Plus he made an incredible difference in her life, when she really needed it.

Remember, you are dealing with real lives and real issues. If you want to retain your clients over the long term, you should become part of their lives. This means that you deal with the issues they encounter in stride without letting the issues get in the way of their training. That may mean going the extra 10 percent, but that's what sets you apart as a trainer.

TRAINING TIP:

You may not have control over the situation that's keeping your client from working out consistently. Find out what it is and go the extra 10 percent if necessary.

POINTS TO REMEMBER:

- There are different ways to motivate clients. The more you know about your clients, the easier it will be to choose motivational techniques that will work for them.

- One of your goals as a trainer it to help your clients develop self-efficacy, so that they believe that they can handle the challenges they encounter in the gym.

- You can't control what happens in your clients' lives, but by keeping their needs in mind and going the extra 10 percent, you can retain them and obtain additional referrals as well.

Chapter 9

The Top 10: Typical Client Types and How to Work with Them

"In the middle of difficulty lies opportunity."

- ALBERT EINSTEIN

As a trainer, you'll find that no two clients are alike. Clients range from shy to intimidating, compliant to easily distracted, and fanatical to undedicated. Each person brings his or her own challenges, issues, and abilities. You've already learned that the more you know about your clients, the easier it is to motivate and work with them.

However, while every client is unique, many fall into 1 of the 10 general categories described in this chapter. Understanding these "types" will help you communicate effectively with clients while reducing the risk of boring, intimidating, or insulting them. Read on for a description of the "top 10" client types and how to work with them.

The Always Off-Track

The Always Off-Track client never focuses on the workout. It's a constant struggle getting Always Off-Tracks to give 100 percent. They do enjoy your company and are happy to chat about whatever pops into their heads. On the bright side, the Always Off-Tracks make time fly as they entertain you with stimulating conversation.

A Real Life Always Off-Track

Justin started training with me after his trainer left our gym. He had worked with this trainer for 8 months but didn't have the results to show for it, which confused me. Justin's previous trainer was qualified and had gotten great results with other clients. I decided to take Justin on as a challenge to figure out what the missing piece of the puzzle was.

Justin and I talked for an hour at our first meeting. Justin was young, athletic and had no injuries. He wanted to put on muscle and seemed committed to his goal. We spoke about his exercise history, goals, and any possible barriers, and nothing jumped out at me as being a problem from that initial conversation.

Justin had already been training, so I outlined a 16-week power routine for him that I thought would translate into a better bodybuilding routine later on. I also gave him some guidance on his eating habits and suggested he eat a bigger breakfast, more protein, and lots of vegetables, among other things.

It wasn't until we started training that I understood Justin's problem. During each break between sets or exercises, he would talk about sports, cars, philosophy, or anything else on his mind for several minutes. I didn't have an issue with this during the anatomical adaptation phase as my goal was to build a strong bond and get his continual buy-in. But as time went on, I realized Justin couldn't focus.

From the minute he walked onto the floor, he wouldn't stop talking. He would even continue his conversation in the middle of his working sets! During his breaks, he wouldn't start his next set until he had finished his point, which would take upwards of 5 minutes.

This created 3 problems. First, his breaks were far too long, so Justin wasn't getting enough of a training effect. Second, I had trouble fitting in his entire workout in the time we had. A young guy who wants to put on weight needs a lot of training volume. I couldn't possibly fit in the requisite amount of work in an hour with all of his talking. But third, and most important, was his lack of focus. He was never fully engaged in his workouts, and lack of focus is detrimental to increasing power.

I decided to apply a version of Pavlov's experiments and train Justin with a beeper. I set my timer to the allotted break time, and when his break was over, it would beep. He would then start his next set, no questions asked. If he didn't comply, I had him do positive punishment— he would do 2 jump squats or 2 plyometric push-ups, depending on whether he was doing upper-body or lower-body exercises. This meant that Justin knew he had to do something immediately when the beep sounded, and the positive punishment helped prepare his body for a set of power lifting.

After a year of training, Justin's squat improved from 95 pounds to 215 pounds and his bench press went from 105 pounds to 190 pounds. He still chats with me about a wide array of interesting subjects before and after workouts, but is 100 percent focused during the actual sessions.

Always Off-Track Challenges

Your biggest challenge with these clients is focus. Your job is to get them results, and they won't get them unless they're engaged in their workouts. Also, if they're not focused on their exercises, you'll have to repeat yourself constantly. Getting Always Off-Track clients to complete their workouts in the allotted time can be a challenge because 45-second breaks inevitably turn into 3 minutes.

Always Off-Tracks often get bored with your workouts since they don't take the time to dive in and understand their purpose. They constantly ask you to change it up. Finally, Always Off-Tracks are often avid readers who want to try every new invention or workout regime. You'll probably find that you spend a lot of your time at the beginning of sessions debating the latest fitness trend.

Always Off-Track Solutions

Training Always Off-Track clients often takes a little creativity. Your goal is to figure out a way to improve their focus *without losing sight of their goals*. Using a stopwatch, like I did with Justin, works well. Say something like, "When you hear the beep, you go!" Positive punishments for non-compliance such as "burpees" work well if your client wants to burn fat.

Sometimes all it takes is sitting the client down, revaluating his goals, and making sure that he buys in to the program. If I think an Always Off-Track client is always talking because he doesn't know what he should be doing during breaks, I'll explain the importance of mentally gearing up for the next exercise between sets.

If you suspect your client is bored, make sure that you explain your workouts, progressions, and vision to your client. Boredom stems from a lack of understanding on your client's part. When you explain what to look for, they'll be motivated by small improvements.

Content Kathy

The typical Content Kathy has had an injury or loss of function, and because of that, she's happy just to be exercising again. Or she may be an older client whose primary goal is to maintain her ability to get around. Content Kathys usually don't care about progression or lifting heavy weights. Most of them prefer lower-key workouts that include lots of stretching.

A Real-Life Content Kathy

Leslie came to me with a whole host of injuries. She had copies of her MRI that revealed a herniated disk, and she had a doctor's note stating that she suffered from patella femoral pain. Leslie also suffered from obsessive-compulsive disorder and asked that I avoid using numbers with her. She refused to let me perform an assessment because she said she would dwell on the results too much.

As you can imagine, setting specific goals for Leslie was out of the question, but I agreed to train Leslie once she got full medical clearance from her physician. Through continuous assessment of her movement patterns, I was able to identify Leslie's imbalances over time. (It took longer than it would have as I had to sneak my assessment in without her noticing.)

I saw Leslie twice a week for 2 years. Leslie was different from any client I'd had before. She didn't need motivation from me as her intrinsic motivation was based on maintaining pain-free function. Yet Leslie was always in a great mood, and she was happy to be active. She loved feeling her body move and wasn't interested in increasing her number of reps or how much she lifted. Yet over time, I was able to challenge her more to help her get stronger.

My work with Leslie helped her retain her function and stay pain-free. She was able to remain active in her everyday life, which was most important to her. And she was able to garden, shovel snow, and carry groceries—things that she hadn't been able to do before! Her goals may have seemed minor compared to some of my clients, but reaching them made her a happy client.

Content Kathy Challenges

Content Kathys often have lots of injuries. Keeping them healthy is your biggest challenge. A second challenge is that the typical Content Kathy loves working out—as long as it's not too challenging. They love feeling their body move but they don't want to strain or push too hard. You have to avoid being lulled into a state of equilibrium when training this client.

Content Kathy Solutions

Every Content Kathy is different, but each needs direction. She's come to you because you have the knowledge to help her. Your job is two-fold: to organize her workouts in a safe, efficient manner, and to subtly push her while making the workouts enjoyable.

The key to dealing with this client is being willing to veer from your usual training model to meet her needs. You must accept that you can't get this client the kind of results that you expect from others because she doesn't want to push that hard. Yes, it can be difficult to accept a client failing to work as hard as *you* think she should. But with Content Kathys, you must remember why they're exercising and what their goals are, and then work within them. In Leslie's case, I couldn't give her specific numbers, but I was still able to help her meet her goals. You can do the same with the Content Kathys you train.

Assiduous Monster

The Assiduous Monster is the hardest working person in the gym, day in and day out. This type of client loves to "feel the burn" on every exercise, and he won't stop until he's given everything he has. He leaves the gym exhausted after every workout, and rarely misses a day of training.

A Real-Life Assiduous Monster

Alex had been doing CrossFit, which includes many high-intensity workouts before training with me. He loved the feeling of exhaustion he got from those workouts, but his assessment revealed a number of muscular imbalances. His hamstrings, hips, calves, and chest muscles were all tight; his lats and glutes had poor activation; and his core strength was almost non-existent. In short, Alex was prepped for disaster.

After going over the results of the assessment with Alex, I told him I wouldn't train him unless we started with an anatomical adaption phase. This would force Alex to take a step back to ensure his safety moving forward. I also laid out my long-plan, which included plenty of high-intensity training when he was ready, and he agreed to the program.

It took 6 full weeks of daily foam rolling, dynamic stretching, and activation exercises to get his body back in order. I also took that time to re-teach him the squat, deadlift, pull-up, and push-up and gave him some nutrition advice.

After those 6 weeks, Alex and I talked again and I gave him my plan for moving forward. By that point, he understood that my job wasn't just to push him as hard as possible, but to help him exercise with proper form so he could get the results he wanted. I developed a list of 18 exercises that would make up our workouts. Each day would be different, but would include lots of high-intensity cardio throughout. I would teach him proper form for each exercise, choose the specific exercises for the next workout, and keep records of reps, weights, and rest periods for each exercise.

This plan gave Alex the variation and the challenge he wanted, but it also let me stay in charge of the workouts. Alex could work out as hard as he wanted, as long as he stayed within the parameters of the program. By training with me, he continued to progress and reach his goals.

Assiduous Monster Challenges

It's difficult to convince Assiduous Monsters to slow down when needed. They feel like they're not getting their money's worth if you don't bring them close to passing out every session. But going all out every workout may eventually lead to injury and in order for progression to happen, you have to program lighter days among the tough ones.

After years of training, the Assiduous Monster may also have bad form and minor injuries and imbalances that must be fixed. A thorough assessment will help you determine how to address these issues.

Assiduous Monster Solutions

These clients have usually participated in exercise programs before, but they probably weren't well-rounded. They may have focused on strength training while ignoring stretching and cardio, for example. Assiduous Monsters may not see the value of a personal trainer, so your first step should be to educate them on the benefits of working with somebody who has the requisite knowledge and passion—namely, you.

A full assessment will reveal what the Assiduous Monster needs to work on, so be frank in telling him what needs to be done. By showing him his weak points, you're giving him a challenge, and his personality will have him chomping at the bit to fix his imbalances.

You must take charge when working with Assiduous Monsters. Don't let them dictate their workouts; you're the trainer. Make sure they're aware of why and how your plan is different from what they were doing before, and most of all, that they know how it's going to help them.

If the Assiduous Monster refuses to change his ways after your attempts to educate him, you may want to encourage him to look elsewhere for a trainer. The short-term gain of training the Assiduous Monster is not worth hurting your reputation, or worse yet, a lawsuit if he gets hurt.

Challenging Charlie

The Challenging Charlie questions everything. These clients are sceptical of you and your gym and won't commit to anything long-term. Whether they've exercised before or not, they've probably done research before hiring you and may want to "test" you early on.

A Real-Life Challenging Charlie

Daniel had been working with a trainer for 18 months before he met me until the studio he trained at closed down. Initially Daniel was stand-offish. He refused an assessment and didn't give detailed answers to any of my questions. After I learned more about his past, though, I realized that he had been poorly trained before. His previous trainer had promised results, but Daniel hadn't achieved them. As a result, Daniel's view of the industry had been tarnished. I had to show him that I was different.

Since Daniel refused an official assessment, I secretly worked the assessment into the first 3 workouts. After each exercise I would take a minute to tell him in detail what was happening in his body. I started to answer his questions before he had a chance to ask them, and as the workouts went on, Daniel gained more faith in me. I trained with him several times a week for 2 months; after that, he felt confident that he had developed a good routine and we parted ways.

Challenging Charlie Challenges

The Challenging Charlie doesn't converse easily. Your questions will be met with one-word answers. They've often done some research before meeting you and want to test you before they commit.

I love it when clients educate themselves, but the problem is that their research isn't always accurate. Setting out a long-term plan for a Challenging Charlie is difficult due to lack of information and commitment. He may stop you midway through your description to remind you that he hasn't signed up for anything yet.

Challenging Charlie Solutions

Because Challenging Charlies have usually had bad experiences in the past, it's important to take your time to educate them about how your approach will be different. Often, educating them about what you're doing, and why, helps convince them of your value.

Before every workout with a Challenging Charlie, I'll take 5 minutes to explain my plan for the day and why I'm doing it. I use the Excitation System often and explain how the exercise will move him closer to his goal. When you take this approach, a Challenging Charlie will develop faith and trust in you.

The Quiet Assassin

Quiet Assassins kick butt! They come in the gym and give you 100 percent every time. It doesn't matter how their day went—and this is convenient because they'll never talk about their day. The typical Quiet Assassin never speaks about anything other than the workouts and, even then, words are few and far between. Getting to know Quiet Assassins (or even gathering information about their work, family, or social life) is like pulling teeth. (With luck, over time the client will become more comfortable and become an Assiduous Monster.)

A Real-Life Quiet Assassin

My client, Lin, was a 28-year-old engineer who had been working with another trainer at the club. Besides her exercise history I knew little about her life, other than the fact she had two parents and a sister who got married midway through her training. (I only knew about her sister because she told me about the wedding 2 days before she took a week off from training.)

I've never had a client who worked harder than Lin, but she said little during our sessions. I spoke a lot during the workouts, giving her instruction and background information on the exercises, and shared anecdotes to break the silence. Lin's response was always a nod and occasionally, a smile.

After training her 2 times a week for a full year, Lin gave me a holiday card that surprised me. She poured her heart out in that card, and thanked me for getting her through a really hard time in her career and personal life. She said that she always looked forward to the quiet motivation and Zen-like atmosphere of our workouts and thanked me for my professionalism and knowledge.

Lin had been listening all along. After that first year, Lin's demeanour changed. She still worked her butt off but spoke with me during breaks. She seemed more comfortable than she had been before, and continued to train with me until I left the gym to work at our new facility.

To this day, I don't know what was going on in Lin's life. I admit it was none of my business! My job was to give Lin a great workout every time. I provided her with a service and if she wanted it to be silent, I had to accept that. I still did my job and described my short- and long-term plans to make sure we were on the same page. I also spent the time and detailed the importance of her exercises. But it was only later that I discovered I had made a difference—she was simply too mentally drained from her personal life to interact with me.

Quiet Assassin Challenges

It's hard to gather information about the Quiet Assassin, which makes establishing a relationship difficult. Every workout is like a bad first date. You will receive one-word answers to every question that you ask the Quiet Assassin, and he probably won't ever ask anything about you.

Since you never quite know where the Quiet Assassin's head is, programming in long-term progression is difficult. They may not tell you how long they want to train with you and getting a grasp on the Quiet Assassin's goals can also be tough. As a result, you may struggle with designing your workout sessions. In addition, any scheduled rest periods often consist of awkward silences broken only by one-word answers to your questions. Quiet Assassins make you second-guess yourself, and they're hard to retain as clients because of the difficulty in creating a solid bond with them.

Quiet Assassin Solutions

The best advice that I can give when dealing with arguably the most challenging client type is this: "stay the course." Quiet Assassins often have issues that they're dealing with and see the gym as an oasis. It's important for you, as their trainer, to not get offended when they don't share any information about their personal lives with you. Your job is to give them great workouts and to educate them. Don't get frustrated about the lack of feedback you may get; focus on challenging them in the gym to keep them coming back.

Keep in mind that once they've battled through their personal issues, Quiet Assassins may eventually open up to you. Then you may find out that they're grateful for the help you've given them. At that stage, they're likely to remain loyal clients.

Know-it-All

Initially the Know-it-All may be your most challenging client. He's probably been exercising for years and will tell you that he just wants a program to follow. He's convinced that he can already perform all of the exercises and won't need to spend much time with you. He'll often give one-word answers to your questions and he will seem closed off to conversation. Know-it-Alls usually don't seek a trainer on their own but are referred to me by a friend or family member.

A Real-Life Know-it-All

Phil came to me after I trained his daughter before her wedding. She'd bought her parents an introductory pack of training sessions, but warned me that her dad would be a challenge to work with. Phil had been active his entire life. Now retired, he did 3 days of weights and 1 or 2 days of light aerobic activity each week despite having sciatic pain, knee pain, and shoulder pain and stiffness.

I was prepared for Phil to be a Know-it-All because his daughter had told me he'd be more interested in showing me what he already does than listening to my instruction. And Phil was, by definition, a Know-it-All. He hardly let me introduce myself before giving me a complete run down of his self-prescribed program. I let him speak but took careful notes so that I could refer to them later.

Once Phil was done, I did an assessment so I could gather as much information as possible before attempting to correct his faults. The assessment showed that Phil suffered from numerous imbalances in addition to pre-diagnosed arthritic pain in his knees and left shoulder. His lower back pain seemed to be a result of hip immobility, which had been worsened by doing hundreds of crunches every day he worked out.

After his assessment, I sat down with Phil. I first laid out the positives in his self-prescribed workout. After "pumping his ego" a bit, I went into detail about his lack of mobility and why it was causing him pain. Finally, I congratulated him on staying active throughout the years and into his retirement.

This is called the "sandwich" technique. In short, it's sandwiching the trait you want to change between two things that the trainee already does well. I told Phil that I wanted to spend the entire first hour making him comfortable with a full dynamic stretching routine that he was to do before exercise. I didn't think he was happy about it, but he agreed.

I must have asked Phil 20 times throughout his first workout how he felt. I wanted to make the sensation of stretching emotional for him so that he could connect to it later. After the first workout, I could tell that Phil was reluctant to continue. To my surprise, when he came back 3 days later he had completed the prescribed warm-up before we met.

I took 10 minutes to explain the initial anatomical adaptation phase, and Phil immediately started to fit his self-prescribed workout into my initial phase. He was trying to prove his worth by showing that he had developed a similar program, so I decided to utilize a different method. I told him the name of each exercise, and asked him to show it to me. If he didn't know what it was, mission accomplished! He was now ready for me to teach it to him start to finish.

If he did know the exercise, I used the sandwich technique to pick out an aspect of the exercise that Phil executed well. I then gave him a suggestion, and finally, added another aspect that he was doing well. For example, on the squat, I noted that his heels stayed down. I then told him to keep his shoulders back and lower himself down in a more controlled manner, and added that his breathing was good.

Phil's biggest problem was his pride. He had been working out for 45 years, so what could a 24-year-old trainer teach him? My goal was to gain his respect, which gave him a reason to listen to me. During the first session, I made him listen to my explanation on the importance of stretching and spent a full hour teaching him the proper form. That initial hour established a clear line of authority that, up until that point, wasn't there. In our second session, I showed him that I valued his knowledge but wasn't afraid to correct him when necessary.

After our initial 3 sessions, Phil bought a package of 10 more on his own. He still wanted to design his own program, but now he knew he needed some help. It may not have been a perfect solution, but at least Phil realized the importance of my coaching and we were able to work together.

Know-it-All Challenges

The Know-it-All usually comes to you because of someone else, not because he really wants to train with you. He may not view you as an authority or respect your knowledge, and therefore he's less likely to listen to what you have to say. I've found that Know-it-Alls are more interested in showing *me* how they do things before I attempt to instruct them.

You also don't have much time to make an impression with Know-it-Alls; their attention span is short and they probably don't see the value in the initial meeting. Most of the time, they'll only come for a session or 2, which means you have to educate them on your value during that time.

Know-it-All Solutions

Keep in mind that Know-it-Alls aren't trying to be rude or disrespectful. They just don't see the value in training with you, so you have to prove yourself. Always listen to what the Know-it-All tells you before trying to sell him on your system. Second, make sure that you establish yourself as the authority figure. Show him that you're not afraid to seize control and gain his respect. Third, make sure that you ask for his opinions and make him an integral part of the training process. When you reiterate the good points of his previous work, he'll often want to address his weaknesses.

Apathetic Anne

Apathetic Anne is uncomfortable in the gym and usually doesn't want to be there in the first place. Like the Know-it-All, Apathetic Anne probably came to you not of her own volition, but either because her family pushed her to exercise or her doctors suggested it. Apathetic Annes are usually shy and reluctant to divulge too much information to you.

They also don't want to spend one more second in the gym than they have to.

A Real-Life Apathetic Anne

Remember Cindy and Pam from chapter 5? Helen was one of the clients they referred to me. Helen's doctor had repeatedly advised her to start an exercise program since she had severe chronic low back pain, had osteopenia, and had low energy, which was possibly due to abnormally low blood pressure.

When Helen finally came in, my primary goal for our initial meeting was to make her feel comfortable. I'd already spoken to our receptionist and asked her to make sure to greet Helen and make small talk with her when she came in. When I sat down with her a few minutes later, we spoke in detail about her medical history and concerns. I then told her about my background, using examples of people I'd helped who had similar issues. I took her on a tour of our facility so she would know where everything was.

Helen agreed to meet me once a week, but would only commit to 3 sessions up front. Those 3 sessions turned into 10. When she completed those, she bought another pack of 20 sessions, and next, 50 sessions! After all her hard work, Helen's serious back pain disappeared and she regained her overall strength. She loves coming into the gym now and will stay to chat with the receptionist for 20 minutes before leaving.

What worked with Helen was making sure the gym was a place where she would receive gentle encouragement in a comfortable, non-intimidating environment. As she progressed, Helen gained not only strength, but also confidence and self-efficacy. She is now a dedicated exerciser and client.

Apathetic Anne Challenges

There are two main challenges with an Apathetic Anne. First, she is probably uncomfortable at the gym. Second, this client is almost always a beginner and has little or no exercise experience.

Apathetic Anne Solutions

When you encounter an Apathetic Anne, remember to step back and focus on making her feel comfortable. She probably hasn't come to a gym before because of the intimidation factor. When you first meet this client, make sure to listen to her carefully and start the workouts in a private space. Tell her a little bit about yourself to help her connect with you on a more personal basis. When you focus on making her feel comfortable, she'll gain confidence and may turn into a long-time client.

Alison Averse

The Alison Averse client has never enjoyed exercise. Alison Averses are likely to have tried (and failed) a number of different exercise programs in the past. They may have previously worked with a trainer, taken group exercise classes, or tried the latest fad programs in the past, but nothing has worked for them.

A Real-life Alison Averse

Ruth had tried working out on 3 occasions before we met. She had first joined a gym 15 years prior, but quit training after 3 months due to family issues. Five years after that, she joined another gym and signed up for an exercise class where she tweaked her back. She was immobilized for 2 days. Needless to say, she didn't continue. Then, 2 years later, she tried a local Curves chain but didn't stick with it.

When our new Body + Soul Fitness branch opened near her house, she decided to give exercise another try. She was motivated and open to suggestions. She wanted results and trusted that I would help her get them. However, Ruth had developed a number of bad habits through her previous gym experiences. After her assessment, I told her I wanted to be extra careful to ensure proper form and activation before we progressed. I didn't give Ruth a timeline, but I did tell her that I'd give her homework and if she completed it diligently, she'd progress quickly.

It took 6 quick weeks to groove her motor patterns well enough that I felt comfortable pushing Ruth. After that, she progressed quickly. She started a power program and she picked up exercises like the deadlift, clean and press, and squat well. Today, Ruth is still working out 6 days/week and has surpassed all of her original fitness goals!

Alison Averse Challenges

The typical Alison Averse is usually open to suggestions from you. Because she's failed in the past, she may realize that she needs help to get in shape. However, most Alison Averses have bad exercise or eating habits. One of the things you'll want to communicate to an Alison Averse is the value of correcting bad habits before she can progress.

Alison Averse Solutions

The key point in dealing with an Alison Averse is establishing trust. Laying out a long-term plan with the Alison Averse also helps create motivation. Because she's fallen off of the wagon before, this helps her feel confident she'll be able to stick with a program.

Aerobics Alice

The Aerobics Alice doesn't care about form. She wants to look good and *feel* each workout, but she's not interested in detailed explanations of exercises, workouts, or the physiology behind them. The Aerobics Alice has already been active by taking exercise classes or working out with friends. She'll typically see you as a tool for quicker results and will hold you accountable if she doesn't get them.

A Real-Life Aerobics Alice

Rebecca had been training in our gym for a while before I started to work with her. She had just had her third child in 4 years; her upper body was relatively strong but her legs and core were weak. After speaking with me, she agreed to an initial 5 sessions.

I told Rebecca that I wanted to focus on her posterior chain and rebuild her pelvic floor. After the first 2 sessions, Rebecca mentioned that she wanted the workouts to be faster-paced. I made the mistake of pretending not to hear, and continued training her the same way. But when the initial 5 sessions were up, Rebecca didn't want to continue training with me. I did chat with her when I saw her at the gym, and complimented her when I saw her doing the leg exercises I'd given her.

To my surprise, Rebecca approached me again 2 months later. She said she wanted to train more seriously, but I took a hard stance by only agreeing to train her if she committed to a minimum of sessions. After I laid out my plan, she agreed—and the results were mind-blowing!

Rebecca had a strong training base and now I had her commitment. In addition, Rebecca was willing to train 6 times a week. I saw her twice a week and made sure that she was following my program the other 4 days. Within a month, Rebecca was accepting compliments left, right, and center concerning her physique.

After she finished her 20 sessions, Rebecca couldn't afford to continue working with me. But she went back to group classes armed with an extensive toolkit of exercise knowledge. As a result, she was able to perform the movements properly in the group exercise classes and maintained her fabulous results. I stayed in touch with Rebecca even after she moved to a different facility. After a year, she returned for another 20 sessions with me for an extra push again.

In retrospect, I could have dealt with Rebecca better. I ignored her early comment instead of taking the time to explain myself. I also should have recognized that Rebecca was inevitably going to return to group exercise after the 20 sessions, and I should have prepared her better. Instead of losing Rebecca as a client for a full year, I may have been able to keep her on an irregular but ongoing basis.

Aerobics Alice Challenges

The Aerobics Alice client forces you to walk a fine line. Focus too much on form and you'll lose her, but focus too little on form and she may get injured. Without proper form, progression is impossible, which makes it hard to improve beyond a certain point. This leaves you in a difficult position.

The Aerobics Alice often has bad habits to address as well. It's not uncommon to re-teach exercises weekly. The Aerobics Alice may also want to work out with friends between sessions, which can make it hard for her to stick to a routine. Therefore workout adherence between sessions may be low.

Aerobics Alice Solutions

There are 2 basic approaches to take with a typical Aerobics Alice client. You may want to recognize that your client will go back to group exercise classes or working out with friends, and prepare her for it. Add some aspects of group exercise into your workouts and focus on proper form, and you may be able to keep the client on an irregular but continuing basis, such as once a week or even once a month.

The second approach is to take a hard-line approach. If you think that Aerobics Alice would benefit more from your training than from what she was previously doing, tell her. Just keep in mind that it's her goals that matter, not yours.

If you do take this approach, it has to be an all-or-nothing conversation. You cannot bend on your opinion of the most effective way to train. If she refuses to buy in after you've extolled the benefits of your system, move on. But I've found that often clients respect the hard-line approach because you have their goals in mind and are holding true to your values as a trainer.

Busy Bill

Time is the issue with the Busy Bill. He runs in on his cell phone and rushes out the minute the workout is done. Sometimes during the workout he'll even stop to take a call! This client understands the value of working out and usually wishes that he could be more consistent.

Most Busy Bills have trouble committing to recurring sessions every week, and are lucky to get in 2 workouts in a week. Busy Bills often cancel regularly, and don't know when they can reschedule.

A Real-Life Busy Bill

Ed started training with me when his other trainer left our club. I had always seen him working hard and was excited to take him on as a client. Ed had been working out for years and possessed a wide knowledge of different exercises and had solid form. His previous trainer warned me not to give him my cell phone number, which I thought was odd. After receiving numerous emails and text messages between the hours of 2:00 and 5:00 a.m., I knew why.

My training with Ed started off great. I got him back on track, and laid out a long-term plan for him that he was excited about. The first 3 months went by well. Ed started to monitor his eating, cut down on his alcohol consumption, and diligently completed his cardio. He was losing inches and gaining strength, but then work started to take over Ed's life.

He was involved in a nasty legal battle over a business, and making time for exercise became close to impossible. When he did make it in, his attention was elsewhere. The stress caused him to increase his alcohol consumption, and the gains he had made over the past 3 months disappeared quickly.

I was frustrated, but I wanted Ed to stay active during a difficult time in his life. So, I decided to switch our focus. I gave him 2 simple 30-minute workouts and some homework. Every time he was feeling stressed or overwhelmed, he could come into the gym on his own and complete the workouts. My goal was to make the gym his sanctuary. In the meantime, I cancelled all of our organized sessions and told him to call me if he wanted to book a session.

Ed made it to the gym an average of twice a week during that difficult stage of his life and met with me once every 2 to 3 weeks. This lasted for nearly 5 months before the legal issue was resolved. During that time, he didn't make any progress, but he did continue working out, which was my primary goal.

Busy Bill Challenges

Getting the Busy Bill results is difficult. They work out sporadically so any programmed progression is close to impossible. In addition, because their lives are so busy, stress gets in the way of regular work-outs. The typical Busy Bill's eating habits are usually sub-par and a weakened immune system due to stress may cause frequent illnesses. From a scheduling point of view, he can be frustrating because of the frequent cancellations.

Busy Bill Solutions

First, don't overwhelm a Busy Bill. Busy Bills have enough stress and having another appointment to keep doesn't help. If the stress is due to an acute problem (for example, an important work project), give them space. Keep in touch on a friendly basis but be careful not to bug them.

If your Busy Bill's life is always going to be stressful, there are a couple ways to deal with it. The first is to do a mini-assessment every time the client walks in. His physical and mental state will be a wild card. Some days he will come in relaxed, and excited for a break in his routine. Other days he may be so stressed he can hardly move. It's important to read your Busy Bill and take as much time as needed for an appropriate warm-up and cool-down to let his nervous system recover after working out.

The second way to ensure success in overscheduled clients is to give homework. I'll often advise them to buy a foam roller and mat for their house. Twenty minute of foam rolling, even if it's before bed, will help them feel good when they can't get to the gym and give them something to look forward to.

Finally, if a Busy Bill refuses to leave his cell phone in the change room, I always hold it during the workout. If someone calls, I tell him who it is and ask if he needs to take the call. That way he only answers the important calls, and can let others leave messages.

Meet Your Clients' Needs

Note that this top 10 list is only a sampling of the types of clients you're likely to work with. As you gain experience, you'll probably identify plenty more!

Just remember that the beautiful part of our job is encountering many different people and working with them to achieve their goals! Your job will change based on the needs of your clients, and their goals are your first priority. Sometimes it takes hard work, sometimes creativity, and sometimes you may even be forced to bend—but not break—from your training style. Do whatever is necessary to get results for your clients.

POINTS TO REMEMBER:

- While every client is different, most fall into general categories. Understanding each of those "types" will help you train your clients effectively.

- Listen closely to your clients, and pay attention to their body language when you meet and work with them. They'll help you identify what type of client they are.

- As a trainer, you should be willing to bend your training philosophies without breaking them to help your clients.

Chapter 10

In-house Relations: Working as Part of a Team

"Dealing with people is probably the biggest problem you face, especially if you are in business. Yes, and that is also true if you are a housewife, architect, or engineer."

- DALE CARNEGIE

As a personal trainer, you don't interact with many different people over the course of a day. There are your clients, of course, with whom you'll work either in a 1-on-1 or group setting. Your clients may come and go, but your fellow staff members (your manager, fellow trainers, receptionists, and other employees) change less frequently. It's paramount to get along with your coworkers whether you work in a large club or smaller facility.

The Advantage of Staying Put

Before we talk about developing relationships with coworkers, though, let me share a piece of advice an early mentor gave me: *Find a great gym that you're comfortable in and stay there.*

I have seen many trainers throw away the reputation they've worked hard to build for what they think is a great opportunity at another gym. It then takes them at least 4 to 5 months to build up a new clientele. Remember, a good reputation takes years to develop, and there are no shortcuts!

Take a trainer I used to work with, who had a great reputation. He spent 30-35 hours/week training a solid client base—clients to whom he'd already given free initial sessions. When he was offered a position closer to home to start a training program at a 24-hour fitness facility, and a chance to buy into the business, he took the new job. His plan was to train fewer hours but make up for his loss of training time by taking a cut of the other trainers' pay as a co-owner of the business. However, he had left his dedicated clientele and reputation to start over in a new neighborhood.

He went a full year earning very little money trying to get this business off the ground. However, the new business went bankrupt and the trainer had no choice but to work at a big box gym earning a lower hourly rate than before. He once again had to develop a reputation and regular clients. All in all, it took him 2 full years to fill his schedule from the time he left our club.

You will encounter adversity as a trainer, but it's up to you to rise above it. By staying in one place, your reputation will grow and you'll spend less time selling as people learn who you are. If you're not happy with some aspect of where you work, you're probably better off addressing it than to jump ship to a new gym.

TRAINING TIP:

Stability in the personal training business is essential and shouldn't be sacrificed without carefully considering your options. Make sure an opportunity is worthwhile before giving up your hard-earned clientele and reputation.

Building Relationships with Coworkers

Sometimes trainers focus only on the relationships with their clients, or future clients. Don't make that mistake. When you have good relationships with your coworkers, you'll attract more clients and become more successful overall.

Treat all of your coworkers with respect. You don't have to be close friends with everyone you work with, but little things can make a big difference. For example, I ask all the other staff members at my club if they would like coffee when I'm heading out the door to get some. I don't just ask the manager and the other trainers, but I ask the receptionist as well.

The $2 I spend on a coffee is well worth it. It helps create a strong bond and says, "I respect that you're working hard and I want to thank you." Taking note of important events in your coworkers' lives can also go a long way. For example, two members of the staff at our club are in a band. I attend their shows when they play locally, and promote their music on my various social media outlets. I want to show them that I care about them as individuals and support them in their endeavours. As a result, they go out of their way to support me.

As a trainer, it would be great if all of the trainers you worked with shared your training philosophies and took a similar approach to working with clients, but that's rarely the case. To thrive at your job, you must be able to work with trainers you disagree with or even envy.

The Trainer you Envy

I found myself jealous of other trainers early on in my career, especially those who worked tons of hours and therefore made lots of money. I particularly envied a trainer named Jim, who worked 7 days/week, training 7 to 10 clients/day. Jim didn't have any high-level formal education and, from what I could see, he didn't do anything special on the floor. By my estimation, he was making a six-figure living, plus bonuses—for somebody with no formal education, that's a pretty darn good salary!

Over time, I started to recognize why Jim was so successful. He might not have had any high-level certifications but Jim had a great attitude. In addition to his 25+ years of experience, he always had a smile on his face, and his presence improved the mood in the room.

I made a point to study Jim to learn the secrets to his success. Jim greeted every person (not just his clients) who walked into the studio with a big hello and smile, as well as hugs, high-fives, and handshakes. He remembered specific details about his clients' personal lives. I quickly learned that his ability to develop and maintain relationships had made him so successful.

Jim became a mentor to me and I followed him around for months. He taught me the difference between training and coaching, how to focus my energy to survive days that started at 5 a.m. and ended at 9:00 p.m. When he was with a client, he was always "on" but when he was between clients, he would rest. It may have appeared to me at first that he wasn't doing anything special, but he possessed a skill that most trainers are missing. He was able to coach, and that's how I learned to do the same thing.

If you are jealous of a trainer, study and learn from that person. *Look at successful people, not with jealousy, but with curiosity*. Identify what has made them successful, and apply those skills to your own life. Don't be afraid to ask someone you admire to serve as your mentor. Even if he says no, you can still watch, learn, and employ the techniques he uses in your own training business.

The Trainer you Disagree With

There are many different ways to achieve the same goal, so it's not unusual for you to disagree with coworkers' training methods. How you handle this situation will depend on your position in the gym. If you're a new trainer, often the best course of action is to keep your mouth shut as long as the client isn't in danger.

However, if you feel the client is in danger, you should speak to your manager right away. Unless you're a senior trainer or manager, it's not your place to intervene in another trainer's workouts.

If you feel that you can help the trainer address a problem, approach him privately to ask if he's willing to meet with you for 10 minutes. Most trainers are happy to have you help them fix clients' improper form, for example, if you take a helpful, not insulting approach.

For example, Jack had been a trainer at our club for 5 months. He hadn't been a personal trainer before but had a background in kinesiology and a couple of years of experience in a physiotherapy setting. One day on the floor, I saw Jack instructing a female client on the sumo deadlift. I knew that Jack had never performed the exercise himself (you should never teach an exercise you haven't already performed yourself), so I watched from my office. His client was struggling and he wasn't able to correct her. I immediately knew what the issue was—her grip was too wide and Jack didn't know to tell her to grip the bar inside her legs, not outside of them.

Jack had kept the weight light, and his client's form was good, so I waited until he was finished with the workout. I sent him an email and asked him to meet me the next day to help him with his sumo deadlift instruction. (I was the senior trainer, so I had the authority to book meetings, but I would have asked him to meet me regardless.)

During the meeting, I had Jack watch a couple of YouTube videos of people performing sumo squats correctly so he could see proper form. Jack was happy for the help. He practiced the exercise and the next week, demonstrated the exercise to his client, who was able to perform it properly.

Note that I first made sure that Jack's client was safe. If she had been in any danger, I would have intervened immediately. I then sent Jack a private message and helped him with the form and instruction without telling another trainer or client. This preserved his pride and kept the lines of communication open.

The Trainer you Don't Click With

Finally, you may work with other trainers you don't particularly like. This problem exists in any job and usually the best course of action is to keep your mouth shut.

The reality of personal training is that you don't have to have much, if any, personal interaction with the other trainers. You can go into the gym, meet your clients, train them, and leave. The only interaction that you may have on a daily basis is working around each other on the gym floor. Treat every trainer with respect, but if you really don't care for someone, just stay out of the person's way as much as you can. You needn't make small talk or be buds with all of your fellow trainers. Just don't badmouth or gossip about anyone at work—that can turn a personality conflict into a bigger problem.

TRAINING TIP:

You may not agree with, or even like, everyone you work with. But treat everyone with respect, and look for ways to create relationships with your coworkers.

Inside Info – Dean Somerset

Dean Somerset is an international public speaker whose main area of expertise is injury and medical dysfunction management through optimally designed exercise programs. He is also the medical and rehabilitation coordinator for World Health Clubs.

Growing up in Western Canada, Dean worked as a sous chef, delivered pizzas, and had the biggest paper route in town (his words, not mine). Dean studied kinesiology with the intention of becoming a physiotherapist. After 3 years of kinesiology, he realized he wanted to work with the full gambit of clients and decided to become a personal trainer.

After completing his degree, Dean worked as an independent trainer for two years out of community centers and people's houses. For the last 7 years he's worked in a commercial facility primarily with injury rehabilitation and medical management clients.

Dean markets through third party endorsements, mostly referrals from medical professionals, and previous clients. He also maintains a popular blog.

Dean's 3 keys to succeeding as a personal trainer are:

1. Take care of yourself – You're no good to anyone if you run around like a chicken with its head cut off and wind up burning yourself out. Your quality will decrease as the quantity of your sessions increases. Take time to make sure you work out, rest, eat, and de-load your stresses regularly.

2. "Sales" shouldn't be a scary word – Every professional service available has a fee associated with its delivery, and personal training should be no different. Build the value far beyond the cost and you will never have to worry about people objecting to spending money on you and what you can do for them.

3. Always learn and implement – The ability to transfer knowledge to your clients is the essence of training. It will help to empower them to take ownership of their fitness program and make you incredibly invaluable to them as a part of their health care team. If you know more about something than any other trainer and you put it into action, you will get better results for your clients, which will translate into more referrals and a bigger bank account.

Dean's words to live by:

"If you care about this profession, show it. You have to treat it like a business, which means staying organized with scheduling, marketing, programs, invoicing, and taking care of yourself along the way. Take regular vacations, get hobbies, and make sure you live a balanced life."

Dean Somerset is a personal trainer, kinesiologist and the Medical and Rehabilitation Coordinator for World Health Clubs. He maintains a blog at www.deansomerset.com

Managing your Manager

In chapter 2, you learned about what to look for when searching for a job. If you're lucky, you'll wind up with a manager you can work well with, but you may not have control over who winds up managing you. If you have the opportunity to choose, however, the key qualities to look for include:

- **Empathy**. A good manager has been a trainer herself and remembers the challenges of it.
- **Understanding of clients' needs**. A good manager knows who the members of the club are, what they want and need, and how to design appropriate workouts for them.
- **Time management skills**. Meetings are essential but can also be huge time-wasters. A good manager respects your time and is prepared for meetings.
- **Personal connection**. Ideally, you'll have a positive relationship with your manager and legitimately enjoy spending time with her.
- **Leadership**. A good manager is comfortable being the figurehead of the club, and gets along with all of the members there.

While trainers often focus on the negative aspects of their managers, you can always work to improve your relationship with yours. Remember that it's in your manager's best interest for you to succeed, and keep these strategies in mind.

Identify His Style

Understanding how your boss likes to manage is essential for a good relationship. Maybe your manager is hands-on and open to conversation all the time. Or maybe he prefers to keep set appointment times in their schedule and does not appreciate guests outside of those times. Know how your manager prefers to communicate—whether in person, on the phone, or through internal or email messages. If you're not sure about his preference, ask him.

Build Trust

Every good relationship is grounded in trust. Managers are no different. Always do what you say you will do in the time given. If you don't finish a task, be honest. Lying or making excuses will only make the situation worse. If you've made a mistake, tell your boss immediately and start trouble-shooting. He should never feel as if you are hiding something from him.

The second aspect of trust is to avoid blindsiding your boss. Anything negative you have to say about your workplace should be said directly to him. If your manager finds out that you were speaking negatively about an aspect of the business or if he sees that you are seeking other opportunities, it's likely to hurt your relationship with him.

Understand His Goals

Your priorities matter to you, not your boss. Recognize what his goals are and make it known that you are working to help him achieve them. Tell him you want to train 25 hours a week, not to achieve *your* goals, but because the club has set a goal of 1000 hours of training this month.

It's likely your boss has both skills and weaknesses. If you can identify a weakness in your boss' skill set in an area you're knowledgeable about, offer to help. Perhaps your boss doesn't have much experience in post-rehabilitation training for the knee and you are strong in that area. Why not write up a proposal to your manager offering a workshop to your fellow trainers?

Communicate your *Goals*

We've talked about your manager's goals, but what about yours? Your manager should know what your goals are, too. For example, if you're training the number of hours you want to, and your manager is pushing you to sell more, talk to him to make sure he understands your goals. But keep in mind that your manager's job is to challenge you.

If you are training your desired number of hours, consider ways to make your time more valuable. That may mean developing a specialty, pursuing an additional certification, or offering to take on additional projects for your boss. However, if management seems to want you to train more than you would prefer, you may want to consider whether your goals align with the company's.

On the other hand, if you're not training as much as you want, ask your manager to help you develop a plan to get more clients. That might include canvassing the gym, making phone calls, establishing an Internet presence, or creating relationships in the community. When you set goals that have your manager's buy-in, meeting them will make him happy too.

Ask for Feedback

Asking for feedback is one of the most powerful ways to develop a positive relationship. In so doing, your manager immediately assumes the role of not only your boss, but he becomes your mentor as well. Ask for a weekly or biweekly meeting with your boss, and come prepared with pre-written questions or points to discuss.

Be Professional

You'll make your manager happy if you take a professional approach to your work. Your clothing should identify you as a personal trainer. Some gyms require uniforms while others have color guidelines (such as wearing all black or a red shirt and black pants). Regardless of what you wear, you should always have clean, new-looking indoor sneakers and nice-looking athletic pants/shorts or khakis, and a collared shirt or nice-looking athletic shirt. Your clients should know instantly that you are a personal trainer.

Remember that some people still think of trainers as rep-counters, not professionals. Combat that idea by presenting yourself as a well-spoken individual. You needn't quote poetry, but make sure you sound intelligent! Speak slowly and clearly, avoid slang, and listen carefully to your clients when they speak. Even if your clients use slang or improper language, don't follow suit; you never know who might be listening. And never talk about other clients during a session, unless you're sharing a motivating story that you know will help your current client.

During a training session, focus on the client you're training. It's fine to wave or say, "hello" to a client or member during a break in your client's workout, but I suggest you avoid making eye contact when your client is performing a set. Don't let yourself be drawn into a conversation with someone else while you're with a client. If you must, glance at your watch, or motion to the clock and say, "break's up, let's go" to your client, or offer to talk to the person after you're finished with your client.

Make Your Boss Feel Valued

Finally, remember that everybody is human. Everyone likes to receive sincere compliments. Providing positive recognition to your boss about something he does well makes him feel valued and helps you focus on his positive aspects. For example, if your boss hires a new trainer make sure to congratulate him and tell him you're looking forward to working and growing with the new employee. I can tell you from experience that hiring and staffing a club is the most difficult, time-consuming, and second-guessed aspect of any manager's job.

I've learned a lot from the various managers I've worked with and you can do the same. Be open to criticism, and strive to help your manager succeed. By doing so, you'll become invaluable to him and to your gym.

TRAINING TIP:

You and your manager need each other to succeed. Figure out what he wants and needs from you, and strive to give it to him. When you help him reach his goals, you'll help yourself as well.

Is Management for You?

This is a book about succeeding as a personal trainer, not as a manager of personal trainers. But if you're considering taking on a position as a manager, consider whether it's the right fit—and the right time—for you to do so. According to one of my mentors, you're ready to become a manager when you're ready to celebrate other people's successes. Do you already help team members develop themselves? Are you willing to continue to grow yourself, and to take the time to learn to become a successful manager?

I made the mistake of transitioning to management too early. I'd been working as a trainer at Body + Soul's new location for about a year when I was promoted to senior trainer. Initially I was excited! I admit that what got me most excited about the position was the title. After only 2.5 years working in a gym, I was able to call myself "senior trainer" on my resume. I was so clouded by the opportunity of a promotion that I didn't stop to think for a minute what my new responsibilities were. I was being asked to comment on other trainers' etiquette, to offer my opinion on their training style, and to help new trainers develop their business skills. I was also asked to give my opinion on the new location's direction. I was happy to put in my 2 cents, but I really had nothing to base my decisions on!

As a senior trainer, I was also given access to more detailed information on the day-to-day duties of running a gym, and I had a chance to get a front row seat and watch how a fitness club was run. I put fitness education on the back burner for the time being and focused more on learning the sales and marketing part of the business as well as managing the younger trainers.

I stuck with the senior trainer position for just under 2 years, but I can say now that I wasn't an effective manager. There were a number of projects that I undertook which never came to fruition and I was nervous approaching the trainers if I wasn't happy with them. My age felt like a stumbling block since there were times when I was the youngest trainer by 4 years in the club and yet, I was their senior.

Eventually I realized that I really wanted to focus on personal training, and my manager, Jason, agreed that my strengths were in education, not management. I retained the senior trainer title but my responsibilities shifted and my role is now more focused on education and support of trainers rather than overseeing them. That position is a great fit for my background and skills, and I'm much happier now than I was before.

My point is that every manager position may require different responsibilities. To succeed in management, though, consider whether you possess the following:

- **Strong relationships**. To be a manager, you must always search for the truth. To do so, you need to have information sources outside of the regular chain of command. Having good relationships with the people you work with (including receptionists and support staff) and club members is essential.
- **Empathy**. The best managers can put themselves in their employees' shoes. It helps if you have worked various jobs within the organisation before. Empathy is paramount to your success.
- **Listening skills**. The best managers are those who listen to their employees. If you're able to listen to coworkers and consider their ideas in addition to your own, you're one step closer to being a good manager.
- **Delegation skills**. The best managers are able to break down large projects and responsibilities and delegate tasks to others. Make sure you're able to do so; you cannot do everything yourself as a manager.
- **Ability to lead by example**. If you want your trainers to work hard, you must work hard as well. If you're a dedicated, driven trainer who takes your career seriously, you're more likely to succeed in a managerial role.
- **Organizational skills**. To succeed as a trainer, you have to be able to maintain client records, remember information, and stay

on top of what's happening with dozens of clients. As a manager, your duties are doubled (if not tripled), and organizational skills are a must.

Often management positions are offered to those who excel as trainers, and that's likely to happen to you if you follow the advice in this book. Don't jump at a management position until you're ready for it, though. Make sure you have the skills you need, and a supportive team as well before you take that leap. [In the next chapter, you'll learn more about how to ask for a promotion.] Also make sure that you understand exactly what your new responsibilities entail, how much you'll be paid, and how many hours you'll be spending at the gym. You may find that a better title doesn't necessarily translate to a better job.

TRAINING TIP:

Successful trainers are often offered manager positions, but this promotion isn't for everyone. Make sure that you know what's expected of you, and that you have the necessary skills to succeed in that role, before you accept a promotion to management.

Is it Time to Go?

Yes, this chapter started with excellent advice—find a great gym to work at and stay there. However, it's unlikely that you'll spend your entire career at one place. There are a number of different reasons why you might want to change jobs.

Maybe you've outgrown your facility. Say you've switched gears in terms of training, and your current gym can't provide you with the equipment for your newfound training focus. Robert, a fellow trainer, used to work at a boutique-style gym with lots of machines and very little open space. As Robert's training style matured, he realized that he enjoyed powerlifting so he moved to a gym that had Olympic lifting equipment.

You may also outgrow your current facility if you want to move up in the industry. Maybe you want to move into management and there's no room for you at your current gym. Or maybe you want to make more money and your gym pays you a lower salary than you think you're worth.

Another factor is that many smaller clubs are being bought out by large organisations. Trainers will often leave after a take-over whether it's due to new management, a cut in pay, or because they prefer to work for a small neighbourhood club, not a large corporation.

Of course there are other reasons to change jobs, too. You may want to move into management to maintain more consistent hours, or decide to relocate. Or you may find that an opportunity comes along that is a better fit for you and your overall goals. Just make sure that you compare the advantages and drawbacks of staying put versus taking a new position *before* you move on.

POINTS TO REMEMBER:

- Treat all of your coworkers with respect and support them in their work.
- Strive for a positive, open relationship with your manager and make sure that each of you understands the other's goals. Your success is tied to his success, and vice-versa.
- Consider your skills and the pros and cons of a managerial position before you accept a promotion.

Section 3

Growing Your
Personal Training Business

Chapter 11

Get More Green: Making More Money as a Trainer

"I have a problem with too much money. I can't reinvest it fast enough, and because I reinvest it, more money comes in. Yes, the rich do get richer."

- ROBERT KIYOSAKI

While you got into training because you had a passion for it, I'm sure you'd like to make a decent living pursing the work you love. In this chapter, you'll learn about how to make more money as a trainer, regardless of where you work.

The pay range for personal trainers can range greatly depending on the socioeconomics of a gym's neighbourhood and a trainer's qualifications. Generally trainers who work for a fitness club make a lower annual salary than ones who are successfully self-employed. Canadian stats are hard to locate, but according to recent stats, U.S. personal trainers average about $36,000-39,000/year. Their average hourly wage is about $17/hour.

Keep in mind that these figures represent a wide range in income. The lowest 10 percent of trainers average $17,000 while the highest 90 percent are making more than $63,000/year! That's a huge difference.

Of course what really matters to you is how much you are making. As a new trainer, you may not have a lot of say negotiating your starting salary, but understand your starting salary is just that—a starting point. As you gain experience and increase your value, you can ask for—and get—more money whether you're paid an hourly rate or a salary.

Boosting your Value

The fact is that not all trainers are alike. The more experience and education you have, the more money you're likely to make. Yet a lot of trainers neglect personal development. That's a big mistake.

Even early on, I understood the importance of education, and made it a rule to read for an hour a day, every day, Monday through Friday. (If I wasn't able to do it during the week, I made up the time on weekends.) I read everything from science textbooks to journal articles to training manuals to books on business and sales.

The more I learned from books that I could apply (and did apply) to my work as a trainer, the more successful I became. In fact, my business grew exponentially, and my manager started to groom me for more senior roles at the club—even though I was a relatively young trainer. In addition, I started to train some of the newly hired trainers and I continued to gain respect from the people I worked with—all because I took the time to educate myself and continued to learn.

Today at any given time, I am typically reading 2 books—one on a training-related topic and one on a business-related subject. The more I learn about each, the more knowledgeable and marketable I am. That makes me valuable to my employer and to my clients.

Nothing in this world can replace education. It's up to you to take advantage of the fabulous wealth of resources available. You must catch, cradle and use the power that education gives you for a successful career.

TRAINING TIP:

Continue to read, learn, and educate yourself to boost your value both to your employer and your clients. Remember that educating yourself about business, as well as training, will help you become successful.

The next step of boosting your value is getting your employer to recognize it. It's relatively simple to do this—make yourself indispensable. You want to make your company need you more than you need your company.

I've found one of the best ways to do this is to get to know your clients, and other gym members, on a personal basis. You know that you've done a good job with this when members of your club come to you with complaints or concerns to pass on to management. Not only have you become a trusted person to those members—you've also become a resource for market-level research for your managers. In other words, you can gather information when you're out on the floor that you can share with your bosses.

Another way to demonstrate your value is to offer to serve as a mentor to fellow trainers. (You may want to ask your manager for permission to do this first.) Providing newer trainers with informational coaching sessions provides an extra benefit to the organisation. It also helps create a hierarchy, with you at the top of the pyramid.

You may be surprised to learn that offering consistent, honest feedback also goes a long way to proving your value. Most employees are worried that saying anything negative to a manager will reflect on them, but that's not the case. When you are honest, you make your manager's job easier. All of the managers I've worked for have thanked me for being upfront and candid and giving them information they may not have otherwise been able to access.

When you make your manager's job easier, you prove your value. Do anything in your power to help your manager out. If it means staying later to help clean the club because the regular cleaning person is sick, do it. If it means answering phones while the receptionist is on a coffee break, do it. Showing that you're willing to go above and beyond your assumed duties will set you apart from the other trainers.

Another way to add value to your organisation is to offer a new program or class. You may have specific experience that will translate well into a class. For example, if you played baseball, offer a baseball strength and conditioning class. If you lost a lot of weight during your personal journey, you might offer a class that focuses on weight loss. Market yourself by highlighting your own experiences and detail why *you* are the right person to teach this class.

Your goal in teaching a class like this is to attract new clients (and revenue) to the gym. Take a close look around the club where you work, and consider what type of clients the gym is attracting. Then think about your background and how you might reach people that the club isn't targeting. After you've come up with a class idea and some marketing tactics, talk to your manager about it. This will demonstrate your willingness to give the extra 10 percent that will set you apart from other trainers.

Asking for More Money

In some instances, your employer may recognize how valuable you've become and offer you a raise or promotion (or both!). Most of the time, though, you'll have to ask for it. First, request a meeting with your boss, preferably first thing in the morning, and state that the meeting is about professional development.

Second, prepare. If you're asking for a raise, you should know what your gym (and similar ones) pay trainers with your expertise and experience. If you're asking for a promotion, you should know whether your gym is expanding and which positions may be available. If you want to create a position, you should have a good overview of what that position will look like. For example, you might suggest creating a new position of "continuing education coach" which would make you responsible for all of the workshops and continuing education materials for the other trainers.

Gather all relevant information and statistics for this meeting. How many hours have you trained? What certifications do you have? What "extra" work have you done (for example, mentoring other trainers) that has made your supervisor's job easier?

If you're asking for a promotion, list specific ideas of how you will help the organisation in your new position. Do you want to launch new programs to hit a so-far-untapped clientele? Do you see trainers struggling on the floor and think you can help them? Do you think your supervisor is overwhelmed and a promotion would let you take some work off of her hands? Type up your "pitch," and have it ready to present at the meeting. Finally, brainstorm follow-up questions that your manager may ask so you're ready for them.

During the meeting itself, focus on how you will be able to help the organisation through your aforementioned ideas. List some areas of improvement at your gym, and describe how you would address them to benefit the organisation. Make sure your passion rings through.

Expect some follow-up questions and be prepared to answer them. Don't bring up a specific raise yet—wait for your supervisor to do it. You want to make sure that he comprehends the additional value you bring to the table *before* talking money.

At the end of the meeting, thank your supervisor for his time. If your request for a raise or promotion is denied, ask why. Determine how you can address any weaknesses your manager points out, and continue to do your best work. Chances are that now that you've planted the seed, your manager will pay more attention to the great work you're doing and you're likely to get a raise or promotion next time you ask.

Other Ways to Produce Income

Working by the hour, whether for a club or as a self-employed trainer, you're unlikely to make a 6-figure income. And if you're paid by the hour, time off means no money coming in. (If you're salaried, you may be offered paid vacation and/or holidays.) So it's not surprising that many trainers turn to other sources of income to help boost what they make. You'll find a brief look at some of the ways to produce passive income as a trainer below.

However, let me say something first. Be very careful selecting the products and programs you promote. It takes years to build up a good reputation and seconds to ruin it. *No amount of money is worth risking your reputation!* I get asked daily to embed links onto my sites for as much as $100 a month (for 2 words!) and I say no because I don't know anything about the products being advertised. I have also turned down every opportunity to take part in multi-tier marketing programs because I didn't think the workout or supplement protocol they offered was satisfactory.

Just last month I recommended my client buy a treadmill from a particular fitness store—despite another store having offered me 10 percent commission on the sale. Why? The treadmill at the store that offered me the commission cost 15 percent more! No commission or bonus is worth losing a client over. If you "sell out" a client on a deal like this and the client finds out, I promise that person won't be happy— and he'll spread the word about you.

Blogging

In chapter 3, I encouraged you to consider setting up a blog. A blog is worthwhile for most trainers for several reasons. First, your blog and/

or website acts as a calling card. It makes it easy for clients to pass your name on to others, and for potential clients to determine that you're different from other trainers. Answering questions and sharing the latest fitness research and advice also attracts readers, which can make you more credible, and more valuable to your employer. A blog can also produce extra income in the following ways:

- **Product/affiliate programs**. Affiliate commissions are big business, and you can make up to 75 percent of the purchase price on informational products. This makes for a huge opportunity if you have a trusted voice among readers—they're more likely to buy products you recommend. Almost every major fitness, nutrition, and book company has an affiliate program these days; the easiest to implement are ones like Amazon.com and Perform Better, but these offer relatively low commissions. I suggest you only agree to affiliate commissions for programs or products you personally believe in; your readers and clients should be able to trust your recommendations.
- **Advertising**. Advertising on your blog or Website can also produce some passive income. Google ads are the most common form of online advertising but some companies will pay a monthly or yearly fee for banner ads or links within embedded text on your page. Remember your integrity, though, and don't promote anything you don't personally believe in
- **Writing for pay**. As you gain experience writing your blog, you may also decide to pursue writing for online or print markets. This isn't true passive income as you have to put some time in to marketing your article ideas as well as research and write them, but it can help you build your name and make a little extra money as well. There are hundreds of online and print markets that cover fitness-related topics, so identify possible markets and pitch ideas if you're interested in this route.

- **Internet coaching.** When you have an online following through your blog, you can also offer Internet training services. I know some coaches who take on 5-10 clients at a time who pay $150-250 a month each. This fee covers their programming, unlimited email questions and answers, and a weekly 30-minute phone call. Other coaches offer other programs for long-distance clients. For example, one offers a "lift analysis" where the client sends a video of a particular exercise or lift to the coach who then critiques his form and provides advice on how to improve the exercise.

Supplements

Selling supplements is probably the most common way that trainers make a second income. Supplement companies often offer multi-tier marketing programs to trainers and others in the fitness industry. You pay an annual fee to participate, and then you make money when you sell supplements and when you recruit other trainers and individuals to sell the supplements.

A lot of trainers market supplements, but I have 3 suggestions before you take part in a program like this. First, read the "small print" very carefully. Know what you are committing to before you sign up so you're not surprised by hidden costs and responsibilities.

Second, consider the quality of the products, and only recommend supplements that will actually help your clients. Remember how important your reputation is—you don't want to lose it by trying to make a few extra dollars.

Third, remember that these programs can be time-intensive. Your job is to be a personal trainer, not supplement provider. Your efforts should be focused on helping your clients get fit. If taking part in a multi-tier marketing program means you will lose focus on your training work, then I advise against it. In the long run you will make more becoming the best trainer you can be.

Finally, some trainers buy supplements wholesale from a company and resell them to clients for a higher price. I recommend against this— first, it's probably illegal, depending on where you live, and it also violates the company's rules. The last thing you want is a lawsuit or criminal charge!

Merchandise

Depending on where you work, merchandising is another way to make a couple of extra bucks. You can buy "branded" products like water bottles, gym bags, and T-shirts with your logo on them, and then sell them to clients. If you have a strong online presence, you may want to consider partnering with a T-shirt company that will let you design a logo and sell "on demand," which means you don't have to worry about keeping inventory in stock.

Workshops

As you build a reputation as an expert, you may also be able to give talks or lead workshops for a fee. (If you're interested in this and are new to public speaking, check out your local Toastmasters group to improve your presentation skills.) Once you've gained experience, you can approach a certification agency and offer to lead workshops, or set up your own by advertising to clients, friends, family, and colleagues.

TRAINING TIP:

Personal trainers are trusted, and you can leverage this trust to create other sources of income Just be sure to maintain your integrity as it takes years to build your reputation and just seconds to break it.

Inside Info – Mark Young

Mark Young has 11+ years, over 10 000 hours, of training experience under his belt. He earned his reputation through his training and writing online, and is the creator of the dvd set, *How to Read Fitness Research*.

After 2 years of work at a large gym Mark launched his own business by first renting space in a private gym before starting his own facility with his wife a few years later. He wanted to be his own boss and thought that owning his own space to train in would be an easy path towards financial freedom.

In 2009 Mark and his wife stepped away from ownership to raise a family. He has rented space to train his clients and maintained a kinesiologist position in the Bariatric Medical Program at the Hamilton General Hospital in Ontario, Canada. Currently he is working as a private trainer and maintains a strong following on both Facebook and Twitter.

Mark's 3 keys to succeeding as a personal trainer are:

1. Being good at business – I chose this as number one because if a trainer has any inclination to go out on their own, they MUST have a strong understanding of business. If they do not they'll be buying themselves out of a job rather than buying a business... and I've been there. Develop systems. Plan your marketing funnel. Create call scripts, and upsells. Incorporate. Make sure you have enough capital. If any of this stuff sounds foreign, you'd better learn it before you start. Early mistakes can cost you dearly. Don't get overzealous and rush into anything. Plan carefully.

2. Be good at what you do – Once you've established your business systems, you must establish your training systems and you must keep up to date with industry trends. And along the same vein, don't just follow what you've heard the latest experts are doing. Make sure there is a sound scientific basis for what you do with your clients.

3. Eat well and train – Trainers so sincerely want to help others that they neglect themselves. Don't do that. Take care of yourself. Not only will you look better (which is one reason why people might listen to you), but you will feel better, avoid burnout, and deal with day to day stressors much better.

Mark's words to live by:

"Contact those who are better than you and ask questions. You'll be surprised how many will answer you."

Mark Young is currently a M.Sc. candidate in exercise physiology. He maintains a blog at markyoungtrainingsystems.com and is the creator of How to Read Fitness Research (www.readfitnessresearch.com)

Make Your Time Work for You

Some trainers are paid a flat salary, regardless of the hours they work. Most trainers, however, are paid by the hour, and for actual hours trained. And if you're one of those trainers, I can promise that you will experience ebbs and flows throughout the year.

My third year of training, I decided to chart the hours I billed/week. Here's what my time looked like:

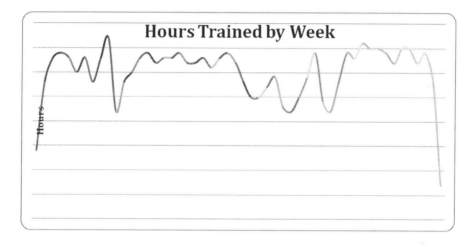

By looking at this chart, I saw that there was serious flux during the year. I was also able to identify several obvious trends. For example, the last week of December and first week of January are pretty dead. In addition, the summer is slower than the other seasons, and March break (March 11-18) was very slow. That tells me that those are good times to plan vacation or other time off.

I was surprised, though, that late-September was one of my slowest times of the year until I examined the demographics of the people I train. Many of them are Jewish, and early to mid-September is when the Jewish high holidays occur. Even though normally this is a busy time for trainers, I have a lot of cancellations during these weeks. From mid-September until Christmas break, though, all Hell breaks loose! This is by far my busiest time so I prepare myself for it.

As you gain experience, I recommend that you complete a graph similar to this for your first 2-3 years of training. It will help you set realistic goals in terms of the number of hours you plan to work. You also may realize that you encounter trends depending on the people you work with. I've found that mid-September is a great time to plan a trip since travel is cheap and I don't lose out on many clients.

I also plan on preparing all of my long-term workout plans and preparing my resources for study during times that I know will be slow. By understanding the demographics of the people I train and my personal ebb and flow, I'm able to reduce the amount of stress in my work.

More isn't Always Better

As a new trainer, you might assume that the more hours you work, the better. That's actually not the case. Yes, as a new trainer, you'll put in extra hours, marketing yourself and getting clients to hire you. But at a certain point, you should reach a level where you're training a number of hours that you can sustain over time.

Two years into my career, I found myself training close to 160 hours/month. I was spending 13- and 14-hour days at the gym to market myself and train clients. At first it seemed like a great idea financially. I was working a ton of hours at what I considered a high hourly rate. But I couldn't sustain the pace. I was working 6-7 days/week and sleeping only 4-5 hours/night.

There was no way that I could give all of my clients the attention they deserve, so I had a high rate of attrition, or client loss. That forced me to spend even more time recruiting clients, and the vicious cycle continued. Finally I took a closer look at what I was actually making. At an hourly rate of $26/hour, and 160 hours/month, I was making $49,920/year. Subtract taxes and the natural ebb and flow of clients over a year and I was actually banking between $30,000 and $35,000/year.

I knew some changes had to happen. I was making myself miserable to put $35,000 in my bank account. I'd quit recreational hockey when I was working 160-hour months. Games were held on Wednesday nights, which meant I had to cancel a night of client appointments to make them. Torn between work and my hobby, I wound up giving up my spot on the team to focus on building my business. I wanted to be the most successful, and therefore busiest, trainer possible.

At the time I didn't realize that being a successful trainer has little to do with being jam-packed busy. In fact, the trainers making the most money are those who have learned to leverage their time effectively. The winter when I quit hockey, I was going through the motions. I woke up at the break of dawn, trained clients all day, and got home with enough energy and time to read for 30 minutes before I fell asleep. I started to contemplate my career because I knew that I couldn't live like I was.

The Block System

After analysing my schedule and my clientele, I found that I had a combination of long-term dedicated clients, program design clients who I saw once in a while, and less dedicated "wishy-washy" clients who scheduled fewer appointments. To work more efficiently, I employed the following steps:

- I first decided the blocks of time that I would train, based on the preferences of my regular, dedicated clients. Those blocks wound up being Monday night, Tuesday night, Wednesday morning to night, Thursday night, Friday morning to mid-afternoon, and Saturday morning to early afternoon.
- I then gave the few dedicated clients who had recurring appointments outside of those blocks of time first dibs on available spots within those blocks.
- If there were any spots left within these blocks, I asked the wishy-washy clients if they wanted to book recurring appointments at open times. If they didn't want to, I suggested they train with another trainer.

- Every time a program design client wanted an appointment, I booked the appointment during a block.

Once in a while I'll go out of my way for a regular client by coming in to the gym outside of the blocks. This is going the extra 10 percent. I now train around 120hrs/month consistently and my retention rate is high.

Yes, I have lost a number of hours where I would have otherwise made money training by blocking off time and politely explaining to clients that I have another commitment. But what I've accomplished by reworking my schedule far outweighs the superficial loss of income.

First off, I got my life back! I no longer wake up at 5:00 a.m. and work until 9:00 p.m. every day of the week. I have time to see friends and family. I also have more time to pursue "passion projects" outside of the gym, like writing this book and creating and running the Personal Training Development Center (www.theptdc.com). I read for pleasure and don't have to miss any important events. I play hockey again and look forward to the weekly games.

But here's the most important aspect from a training perspective. Scheduling my time into blocks gave me more time not only to pursue my personal interests, but to research, learn, and increase my value as a trainer, too.

When I was working 160 hours month, I was making $26/hour, which meant I was earning about $49,920/year. Cutting my hours by a quarter did cut my income by $12,480, true. But that's short-sighted thinking. As a direct result of my revised schedule, I became a happier and more energetic person, I created better workouts for my clients, and I researched and learned more about training. Within a year of my schedule revision, I came close to doubling my salary! Since then, my pay has increased every year while training about 120hours/month.

There is one very simple reason for the continual increase in income: *I do a better job!*

I'm more educated, energetic, have the time to write better workouts, and have the energy to establish stronger relationships with clients. In addition, the money I earn no longer comes solely from training clients. The first year after I made the change to a more efficient schedule, I was promoted to senior trainer and started to earn a base salary plus commissions for referrals. Within 12 months, I was making much more money than I had before, even while working fewer hours.

Here's the point I want you to remember. Instead of training 160 hours/month, collecting my $26/hour salary, and growing more and more burned out, I elected to scale back my hours and make my time more valuable. I used my additional spare time to develop myself and to provide better service to my clients. Management quickly recognized my value, and my hourly salary nearly doubled, even while I worked fewer hours.

Just as important, I was happier in my overall life, and looked forward to sustaining a long-term career in the profession I love. Most trainers don't get into the business because they want to become millionaires, but there's nothing wrong with wanting to make a good living either.

TRAINING TIP:

Consider your long-term earning potential, not just what you're making per-hour. Your number 1 priority, after attracting clients, should be developing yourself and increasing your value.

Getting Started

My suggestion to new trainers is to start with an open schedule. Schedule clients whenever you can, and work your butt off for the first 6 months or so. Then look for trends within your dedicated clientele. Use the block system I described above to organize your schedule in a way that will work for you in the long term.

In the meantime, work on increasing your value. Start researching and developing a specialty that's needed among the people you train. Work on your selling skills and spread the word about your abilities to everyone you meet. In addition, treat every client with respect and focus on developing amazing relationships with everyone you come across. The goal is to turn your clients into your personal "brand ambassadors". They'll be eager to spread the word about how great you are, and you'll be on your way to increasing your income as a trainer.

TRAINING TIP:

To be successful, work on developing yourself and building relationships with the people you encounter. As you increase your value, you'll find that you can increase your income as well.

POINTS TO REMEMBER:

- Educating yourself and increasing your value will help you command a higher salary as a trainer. Focus on what you can make in the future, not only on what you're making right now.

- Always be willing to go the extra 10 percent, not only with clients, but with your coworkers as well. It will position well when you ask for a raise or promotion.

- Once you gain experience, use the block system to work more efficiently and leave time for personal development, education, family, friends, and hobbies.

Chapter 12

Investing in Yourself:
Succeeding as a Trainer

"I was seldom able to see an opportunity until it had ceased to be one."

- MARK TWAIN

So, you've found work as a trainer. You're selling your skills to clients, working with them, and having the satisfaction of helping them reach their goals. So what's next?

That depends on you. Maybe your goal is to stay at your current gym. Maybe you want to change jobs. Or maybe you're thinking about working for yourself. Regardless of your goals, make sure that you invest in yourself to do the best job you can right now—and that you think about your future plans, too.

Avoid Complacency

I compare a trainer's client base to overall fitness level. Once you reach a fairly high level of fitness, it's easy to maintain. It's the same with your client base. I consider a trainer "stable" when he or she is training clients 20 hours/week and developing good relationships with those clients. If you reach that point, and keep doing what you're doing, your client base should stay stable. An inevitable ebb and flow of clients will occur, but referrals should account for any attrition, or loss of clients.

At this stage in your career, your hard work is done—at least for now. I reached this point several years after I started working as a personal trainer. I had put in my time and had given many complimentary sessions. I'd worked with a wide variety of clients and knew whom I was comfortable training. I'd learned how to market myself, and had developed a loyal following. And while the process of education and research never ends, I'd learned enough about different training methods to know how to choose what would work best for my clients.

Yet I found myself at a turning point several years ago. For the first time in 3 years, my numbers were down. I wasn't training as much as I was used to, and I didn't have referrals coming down the pipeline. My client base was dwindling and it had been a long time since I experienced any attrition. Simply put, I was at a loss. I talked to my manager, Jason, about it, and identified the problem. I was bored! I'd been training the same clients for a long time and wasn't being challenged. I'd been coasting, and it reflected on my work.

After taking some time to think about what I *wanted* to be doing (as opposed to what I *was* doing), Jason and I agreed that I would change my senior trainer duties to focus on education and development of trainers instead of some of the other work I wish I had been doing. We devised a new job description for my senior trainer role. I was no longer responsible for day-to-day club operation nor required to attend company meetings. My job was to pick 2-3 trainers each month and work with them individually to enhance their skills.

First, my new role brought me back to what I loved doing. It also forced me to think critically about the programming I was doing for clients. Every time that I worked with a trainer, I remembered all of the creative ideas for effective programming that I used to do. Working with the other trainers forced me to refocus and consider how I wanted to proceed.

I started to re-think the workouts I'd spent so much time writing for my clients and realized that I needed to get back to basics. I had gotten caught up in fancy advanced protocols before my clients were ready. I realized that I needed to get back to the "KISS" (Keep It Simple Stupid) method, and started developing the Focus System.

To start, I sat down with each of my clients and re-evaluated their goals. I then decided on 2 exercises that I wanted them to master—just 2! Usually the exercises were variations of the dead lift, squat, bench press, and chin-up. I then revamped each workout to focus specifically on mastering these lifts. One reason I took this approach was that I realized that beginner clients (and most clients are beginners after all) couldn't master more than 2-3 things at once. Therefore, writing a 3-day split program with 8-10 exercises in each workout was overkill. I shortened my workouts and made them much more specific.

Progression was solely based on these 2 exercises. As long as the client's form was improving or the weight was increasing, I knew the client was making progress. The rest of their workouts consisted of pre-hab, core strengthening, and mobility/flexibility work.

The results of my KISS programming, which I named the Focus System, were astounding. Every one of my clients got great results (I wish I could've said that before) and I once again found myself having to turn away clients. Today, most of my clients now have 2 main exercises per workout that they do for a minimum of 12 weeks. I'm not worried about clients getting bored because they're seeing fantastic results. What I've done is chosen the most important exercises for them at that point in time. I have used the Excitation System to educate them about the exercises and in turn created enthusiasm about their workouts. Once they start to plateau on those exercises, I choose 2 other important exercises and repeat the process.

I realize that linear progressions of this sort won't work forever. But as I said in chapter 1, the majority of personal training clients are in the beginner to intermediate stage of training and this approach is extremely effective. Don't get bogged down by fancy periodization schemes until your clients get to a much more advanced level.

But the real point of this story is to avoid becoming complacent. It's easy to get into a training groove where you're coasting and no longer challenging yourself. But if you don't feel challenged, it may be reflected in how you train your clients.

TRAINING TIP:

Avoid complacency. If you find yourself "coasting," it's a sign you need to change your approach to your business.

Inside Info – Michael Torres

Michael Torres is the owner of Integrated Performance Institute in New York City and a master trainer for Combine360.

Michael began his fitness career as an NCO in the US Army at Fort Bragg. As a team squad leader in an Airborne unit, the health and wellness of his soldiers was a top priority. He led them through tours in Afghanistan and Iraq.

After leaving the army Michael worked on the corporate side of the fitness industry. He was assistant general manager and personal training manager at commercial clubs. He then decided that he wanted to be more directly involved with his clients.

Being a licensed massage therapist and a personal trainer allows him to provide a wide range of services. Michael started Integrated Performance as the sole proprietor. His clients come primarily through referrals, although the gym has an established presence online through their webspace and social media.

Michael's 3 keys to succeeding as a personal trainer are:

1. Personal Training is a "profession" not a job – It takes continued growth and experience as well as dedication

2. Provide results – There is no better way to achieve success in your business. Keeping yourself on top of current research and trends is the best way to get on top and stay there.

3. Educate your clients and empower them to be better – The smarter your clients are the better they will perform. That will lead to greater results and more referrals for you.

Michael's words to live by:

"Continue to learn, however be practical in your education. If you take a course just don't burn through it to add some initials behind your name. Own that material, embrace it; and then move on."

Michael Torres CPT, LMT is the owner of Integreated Performance Institute in addition to being a Master Trainer for Combine360, a Sports Performance Certification powered by Under Armour, Gatorade and IMG Academines.. His website is www.iperformanceinstitute.com

Who Do you Work For?

While many trainers thrive working for an employer, many others want to be their own boss and become self-employed. Your personality will impact which is a better fit for you, but most trainers wind up working as independent contractors (as opposed to employees) whether they work at a gym owned by someone else or not.

As a trainer, I've always been an independent contractor even though I work for an organisation. I'd rather be an independent contractor instead of an employee for several reasons:

- **Scheduling freedom**. You already know that I enjoy traveling. This year alone, I've spent 14 weeks traveling to locales ranging from South Korea to Panama to San Francisco to New York. As an independent contractor, I don't get any paid vacation, but I can plan to take my vacation time during slow training times. I doubt that any employer would let me take 14 weeks of vacation in any given year! I can also set my own schedule and choose which days and which times of day I work.
- **Opportunity for other work**. Many trainers train clients outside of their club or studio. (Just remember that you must declare all of your income, regardless of who pays you!) As an employee, you usually must sign a contract that prohibits you from training clients "on the side." An independent contractor's agreement may require you to work a minimum number of hours, but you're free to train other clients as long as you meet that minimum.
- **Personal/professional projects**. If I were an employee, I wouldn't have had the freedom to schedule blocks of time that enabled me to develop the Personal Trainer Development Center. In addition, my boss could have seen the center as a competing business and forced me to shut it down. If you're like me and have an entrepreneurial mindset, working as an independent contractor gives you the ability to pursue other opportunities or interests.

- **Financial benefits.** Independent contractors are usually paid a higher hourly wage than employees, which makes sense. Since gyms don't pay independent contractors benefits, paid time off, or certain taxes, they can afford to pay these trainers a higher hourly wage than in-house employees. Most trainers have minimal expenses—you invest in items like athletic clothing (you'd probably buy that anyway), a cellular phone (again, you'd need that anyway), and possibly some fitness equipment. You may need to rent studio space, but you can take that as a legitimate tax deduction.

- **Tax benefits.** Depending on where you live, you can write off expenses related to your business that may include a home office, laptop, your Internet connection, workout clothing, books and journals related to fitness, and continuing education. [For more information about the tax implications of working as an independent contractor, check out www.cra.gc.ca if you're a Canadian resident and www.irs.gov if you live in the U.S.]

Of course there are benefits to being an employee as well. Employees enjoy more job security, managerial support, educational opportunities, and often receive benefits (think sick days and paid vacation) that independent contractors do not. Deciding which option is a better fit will depend on your priorities and your opportunities.

TRAINING TIP:

There are advantages and drawbacks to working as either an employee or independent contractor. Make sure you know which one is the right fit for you.

Should you Open your own Business?

Many trainers have a goal of opening their own training business, so I'd like you to consider the following factors before you do so. I caution against opening your own gym right off the bat. Yes, it's tempting, but many trainers struggle for years or go bankrupt because they opened up a gym or studio before they had a complete view of the industry. Take the time to develop yourself first. Spend time in different types of gyms and work with as many different types of clients as you can. Fail, learn from your mistakes, and read everything you can about starting your own training business.

Don't open your gym until you are 100 percent confident in your ability to do so, and you have a network to help you. While I've listed 11 essential steps below, this is only an overview; if you're serious about opening your own business, I suggest you read as much as you can about business ownership, marketing, and management. It will help you identify potential issues and launch a successful business.

Step 1: Find a location.

You must feel a "connection" with the neighbourhood where you set up shop. Just as important, the area should be home to the types of clients with whom you want to work. Sure, some owners open gyms in warehouse districts for lower rents and more space, and hope that their reputation will be enough to encourage clients to travel to them. My personal opinion is, why make it hard on yourself? You can accomplish a lot with a small space and even more if you choose a location near a public park.

You needn't commit to the location yet—in fact, you shouldn't. I have this as step 1 to get you to start thinking about the type of studio you want to open and where you want to work. Passion grows from visualization, and to complete the rest of the steps, you will need lots of passion.

You should be doing your market research. Get stats on the demographics of the area from local government sources. Check out all gyms within a 15-minute drive. Go on tours and do your due diligence. You may even want to join the major gyms for a week or 2 to learn as much as possible about how they operate and how their personal trainers work.

When you write your business plan [see step 3], you'll analyse your competition. Even before that, though, you can compare possible locations with the "Drop Analysis" form shown below.

DROP ANALYSIS

Area Code	Houses	Apartments	Businesses	Total
A1A 1A1	776	1700	342	2818
A1A 1A2	1200	231	12	1443
A1A 1A3	124	1892	512	2528
A1A 1A4	150	3700	57	3907
...				
...				
...				

In Canada, you can obtain information about how many local houses, businesses, and apartments there are in a given postal code to create a "drop analysis" like the one shown above. This helps you determine the density of the area and how many locations you could send advertisements or mailings to. In the U.S., your local chapter of the Chamber of Commerce and the Census Bureau are both great sources for this type of demographic information.

I also suggest you perform a competition and SWOT (Strengths, Weaknesses, Opportunities, Threats) analysis for each of your competitors. [see on next page.] The more information you gather on your competitors, the better.

COMPETITION ANALYSIS

Name	Address	Phone number	Hours of operation	Membership fee	Personal Training fees
ABC Gym	1234 Main St	555-5555	Mon-Fri 6am-10pm Sat 7am-8pm Sun Closed	Monthly - $66 Yearly - $684 ($57/month)	Bronze - $55/hr Silver - $60/hr Gold - $70/hr Platinum - $85/hr
DEF Gym	4321 Main St	123-4567	24hrs/7days per week	Monthly - $68 No yearly option	Outside company provides services (subject to change) $73/hr

The competition analysis gives the "bare bones" essential details of all of the gyms close to your potential location.

EXAMPLE SWOT ANALYSIS

Strengths	Weaknesses	Opportunities	Threats
10 years old (established)	Parking is difficult	Younger clientele so a facility comfortable for the 40-60 market could do well as it will also solve the overcrowded at certain times issue (retirees working out in the middle of the day etc.)	Lots of fast food joints nearby
Clean	Complaints of disorganized management	Offer more personal attention	Expensive property
Good variety of trainers in both experience and expertise	Complaints of overcharging or misprocessing payments	More available equipment	Parking is stressful
Squash courts	Closed Sundays	Provide and open dialogue with members at all times	Very small walking by traffic
Big facility	Big facility		
Juice bar	Overcrowded at busy times		
Big sales staff	Dishonest marketing		

Your SWOT analysis should be as detailed as possible. The idea is that you determine the holes in your competitors armour, and figure out a way to fill those holes.

While you're doing research on possible locations, identify which local businesses have the potential to become business partners. Local businesses can be a fantastic source of referrals. When Body + Soul Fitness opened its new location, management identified neighbourhood "influencers," many of whom were business owners, and offered them free 6-month memberships. Within 2 weeks, the investment paid off through referrals and we're still reaping the benefits.

Step 2: Hire a business manager (optional).

Getting somebody to manage the business side of things frees you up to do what you do best—fitness. However, a business manager is also another expense that will cut into your profits. If you plan to run a small personal training studio, you may not need a business manager. On the other hand, if you have big aspirations and want to grow into a large gym or have multiple locations, having a business manager at the start is imperative.

A business manager's responsibilities may include overseeing the day-to-day business of the club, ordering/stocking retail products, organizing client files, handling payroll and bills, and doing marketing and advertising. A good business manager will help your organisation run more smoothly and can help bring in new business and enhance client relations.

If you hire a business manager, make sure the person has strengths that you lack. For example, if you know little about running a business, you must hire somebody who has good business sense. In addition, every business manager *must* have excellent customer service, organizational, and computer skills. The person you hire must also have good ethics; you're putting your business in his or her hands! To find the right person, consider advertising in trade magazines, networking at professional conferences, and asking clients, friends, and family for recommendations. Make sure you "click" with the person you hire.

Step 3: Create a business plan.

Creating a business plan may take time, but it is definitely worth it. You'll need a detailed business plan if you plan to seek investors or partners, or need to obtain financing. A business plan also:

- Plots a course for you and lets you paint a full picture of what you hope to accomplish;
- Helps you anticipate and plan for problems;
- Helps determine whether your plan is feasible. If it isn't, it can help you identify what areas you must change to make your plan work; and
- Reveals where you need assistance.

Business plans vary in their level of detail, but all include the following 7 sections:

1. **Table of contents.** This allows for easy reading.
2. **Executive summary.** The executive summary is a concise (usually 2 pages) description of the business. It introduces the main areas of the business such as distinctive features, target market, competitive analysis, key marketing strategies, legal issues, supplier summary, management team, financial requirements and projections, equity investment, and owners.
3. **Company profile.** This is a snapshot of the positions in your business and who is involved.
4. **Marketing plan.** This section includes industry trends, service and products offered, target market, and competitive analysis.
5. **Operational plan.** This section includes operating requirements, human resources, and suppliers.
6. **Financial plan.** This section includes start-up costs, a cash-flow statement, income statement, and a balance sheet.
7. **Appendix.** The appendix includes additional relevant information.

Your local chamber of commerce or business bureau may have samples for you, or check out Canada Business (www.canadabusiness.ca) or the U.S.'s Small Business Administration (www.sba.gove) for excellent, free resources.

Step 4: Create a professional team.

You'll need to have a good lawyer and accountant you can rely on. They can save you money, and help protect your interests. To find the right professionals, I recommend first asking friends, family, and colleagues for recommendations. Personal referrals go a long way, and it's a bonus if the professional has worked with clients in the fitness industry before.

If you don't have referrals, make sure you interview a number of law and accounting offices before making your decision. Ask if they've worked with small business clients before. You may want to also ask some business-related questions to see how they answer and interact with you. Choose someone you have a good rapport with and feel that you can trust.

Step 5: Obtain financing (optional).

Depending on your financial situation and the size of your vision, you may need to obtain financing. Armed with a complete business plan, you are free to approach a bank or look for investors. There are many "angel" investor organisations (use the Internet to find local ones) that are eager to invest in small businesses. You may also want to ask friends, family members, and/or clients to consider investing in your business.

Step 6: Hire contractors.

Again, ask for personal recommendations as I have heard countless horror stories of contractors failing to finish the work or doing a sub-par job. If you can't get a referral for a contractor, check out local businesses but be sure to do a thorough interview process. Ask that the contractors you speak to provide you with references; if they can't give you names and phone numbers of previous satisfied clients, move on.

You should have a clear vision of your gym and be able to communicate it clearly to the contractor you hire. A professional should be able to take your plan and lay out a step-by-step procedure for making your vision a physical reality.

Step 7: Purchase equipment.

At this stage, you already know whether you need a wide range of fitness equipment or basic rack of weights and mats. Remember to consider what type of flooring and infrastructure you'll have. A lot of trainers are opting for synthetic turf and reinforced walls as crossFit-type and hard-core gyms are becoming more popular. Fitness equipment companies often offer this type of material and can include it in a package, or your sales rep may get a commission for referring you to a company that provides this material. Make sure you use that fact when negotiating a price for your equipment.

Know what you want and need, and shop around. Compare prices and take note of what deals the company will give you if you continue doing business with them. Fitness equipment is big business and reps earn large commissions, so negotiate the best price you can.

Step 8: Create manuals.

This step is often overlooked, but it essential if you'll have any employees or independent contractors working with you. Your business should have a set of manuals that outline company policies and procedures for receptionists, trainers, and managers. Contact your local small business bureau or chamber of commerce for outlines and templates.

Step 9: Hire staff.

Many personal trainers run one-person operations when they start so staffing isn't an issue. If you are willing to answer the phone, clean toilets, track client appointments, manage accounts payable, and handle all of the other aspects of running your business, then go for it. Otherwise use the same steps you would use to hire a business manager to hire staff.

Step 10: Apply the finishing touches.

This "final" step actually never ends as you will continually be adding equipment whether it's a new shoe rack, framed print, or medicine ball. The finishing touches are what give your facility its unique feel so think carefully about the kind of atmosphere you want to have. If you want a neighbourhood feel, you might hang corkboards with picture frames announcing local events and highlighting clients with a "client of the month" program. If you want a more hard-core feel, you might purchase bodybuilding motivation posters, a good sound system, and have stations for chalk, tires, and chains for weight-lifting.

Don't go overboard with decorations and minor details at the onset. You can always make tweaks to your gym later.

Step 11: Market your business.

Now that your studio is built, staffed, and operations are established, you (or your business manager) can start marketing your services. Hopefully you have already developed a reputation that precedes you and clients are banging down your door for your services. I could dedicate a book to marketing, but the most important point to remember is: *market specifically to the clients you want!*

For example, if you're pursuing older clients, promote your gym as a comfortable, safe environment. If you have built a hard-core training facility, send the message with your advertisements, using more aggressive language and photos that show serious bodybuilding. However you advertise, you may turn off some potential clients, but you're not trying to appeal to everyone—you're trying to target a specific audience. Use the SWOT analysis to your advantage and try to attract the people your competitors are not reaching.

Before you Take the Leap…

Remember, this discussion is only meant to *outline* the steps necessary to open your own business. You should plan to spend months analysing all aspects of opening your own gym before you take that leap. Don't make the mistake of opening a studio without doing all of the upfront work first. With proper preparation, including a detailed market analysis, business plan, and outside professionals on board, your rate of success will be exponentially higher.

Your Career—and Your Life

Last chapter, I explained how employing the Block System made me more productive as a trainer. It also gave me the time I needed for myself to pursue interests like hockey and travel, and helped me avoid burnout.

You may think that spending 12 hours or more in the gym every day will help you succeed as a trainer—and that may be true for the first few months, as you build your business. But you have to have a life outside of the gym, too, and you have to take breaks on a regular basis.

When I'm working, I work hard, but I take plenty of time off—14 weeks of vacation this year and counting! In the bestseller, *The Power of Full Engagement*, authors Jim Loehr and Tony Schwartz describe the process of increasing your work capacity. They apply periodization principles to work efficiency and have found that to produce high-quality work, you must push yourself hard, and then take a full break. As a result, the next time you will be able to push harder and longer. And so on.

Planned vacation time will help you recharge, as will taking breaks throughout the workday. Even a short walk makes a huge difference. For example, there's a large park near my gym. I'll take a 30-minute walk there before I am scheduled to see clients in order to build in some necessary downtime. I come back refreshed and ready to work hard again.

Another way to recharge is by mastering a new skill. Attend a conference, take a class, or educate yourself about an area of fitness about which you know little. Earlier in this chapter, I warned against becoming complacent. If you don't continue to challenge yourself, complacency can lead to burnout. That's one reason I love attending workshops and conferences—I always learn new skills that I later apply to my clients' workouts.

For example, I met a woman who was studying to become a personal trainer when I was creating the Personal Trainer Development Center. Her background was in martial arts, so we negotiated a deal where I would help her become a trainer and she would teach me martial arts-based training. I benefitted by learning an exciting set of skills, and my clients benefited because of the advanced bodyweight techniques I could now incorporate into their training.

Personal training is a fulfilling career, but it's a challenging one, too. You'll be worn down physically and mentally at the end of the day, and motivating clients is tough when your own motivation wanes. To succeed, you should be willing to give the extra 10 percent to your clients, but make sure that you attend to your own needs as well. If you're starting to feel bored, figure out what would light your fire again. If you feel like you're coasting, set a new challenge for yourself. And if you feel like you're starting to get burned out, take time off to recharge.

In chapter 1, I reminded you that *you* are your own best advertisement. In chapter 4, I reminded you that *you* are the product you're selling. Let me now remind you that even if you work for someone else, *you* are in charge of your career and your future. That means continuing to learn, continuing to grow, and continuing to challenge yourself.

I believe that personal training is the best job in the world. You play an integral role in the lives of the clients you train. Through your work, you not only provide motivation and support—you enable people to live longer, healthier, more satisfying and more productive lives.

I can't imagine a better definition of "success." I hope you'll find that your career as a trainer is just as satisfying. My hope is that no matter how tired you are, you end every day with a smile on your face.

POINTS TO REMEMBER:

- You are responsible for your career, and your success.

- Before you decide to open your own studio, take the time to consider the advantages and drawbacks of doing so. The more detailed and thorough your plan is, the more likely your studio is to succeed.

- A fitness certification can help launch your career as a personal trainer, but choose the certification that makes sense for your career.

- Avoid complacency. When you feel continually challenged, it will reflect in your work, and help you avoid burnout.

Afterword

First, I want to congratulate you for discovering and second, for finishing this book. You're already 10 steps ahead of the competition. I love helping personal trainers develop successful careers and want to help you as much as possible but it's impossible to include everything I wanted to in this book.

To assist more personal trainers, I created the Personal Trainer Development Center (www.theptdc.com). The Personal Trainer Development Center features some of the best trainers in our industry, each with different specialities, who are all committed to sharing high-quality information no one else is teaching trainers.

The Website is free to use and benefit from; all you have to do is go to www.theptdc.com and start searching. I encourage you to become an active member of our community, and to sign up for our email list to stay up-to-date. We publish new articles weekly and have an active Q & A section that covers everything fitness-related except exercise prescription.

If you're looking for articles on a particular subject, please search our archives or send me an email at jonathan@theptdc.com. If we don't have an article on the subject, I'll ask someone highly qualified to write one.

Finally, I truly hope you enjoyed this book and want to sincerely thank you for taking the time to read it. If you have questions, comments, or criticisms, or just want to say "hi," I'd be happy to hear from you. I love meeting smart, forward-thinking trainers.

For now, though, that's all. I hope that I've ignited your fire, and that it will continue to burn.

To your unlimited successes,
–Jon Goodman

About the Author

Jon Goodman, CSCS, is the creator and head coach of the Personal Trainer Development Center (www.theptdc.com). He has served as a weight room manager, personal trainer, and senior personal trainer in both University and commercial gyms. For more information about Jon Goodman, go to his Web site at www.jongoodman.ca. He can be reached at jonathan@theptdc.com.

Made in the USA
Lexington, KY
13 October 2013